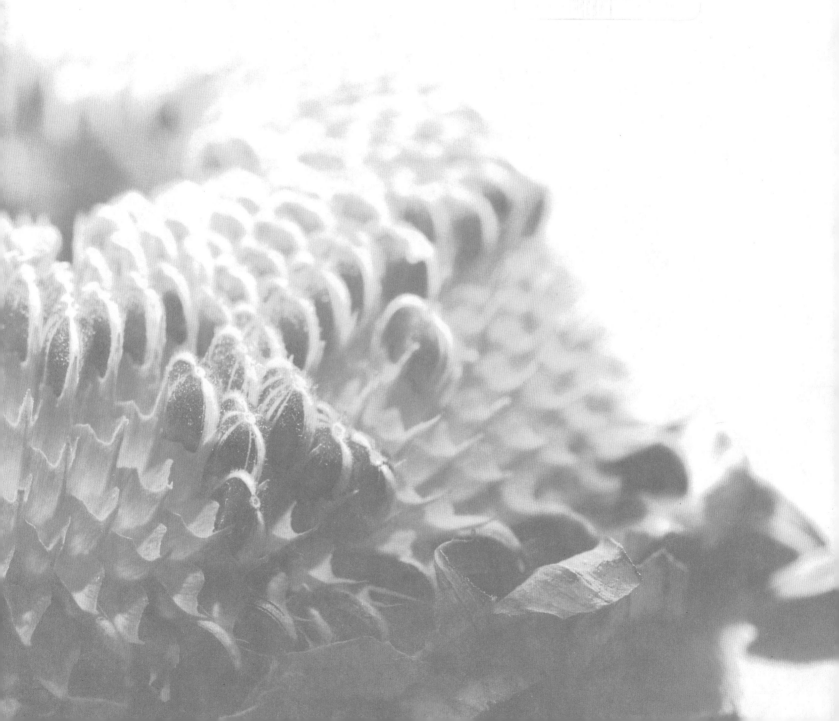

"It is only shallow people who do not judge by appearances. The true mystery of the world is the visible, not the invisible."

OSCAR WILDE

CHIC
SIMPLE ®

BODY

ALFRED A. KNOPF NEW YORK 1994

THIS IS A BORZOI BOOK
PUBLISHED BY ALFRED A. KNOPF, INC.

KIM JOHNSON GROSS   JEFF STONE

WRITTEN BY JUDITH NEWMAN
PHOTOGRAPHS BY KENJI TOMA
STYLED BY JEFFREY MILLER
HAIR AND MAKEUP BY YASUO YOSHIKAWA

DESIGN AND ART DIRECTION BY
ROBERT VALENTINE INCORPORATED
ICON ILLUSTRATION BY ERIC HANSON
TOOLS AND RULER ILLUSTRATIONS BY GREGORY NEMEC
CHAPTER ILLUSTRATIONS BY JEFFREY FISHER

Library of Congress Cataloging-in-Publication Data
Gross, Kim Johnson.
Chic Simple. Body/Kim Johnson Gross, Jeff Stone, and Judith Newman.
p. cm.—(Chic Simple)
ISBN 0-679-43224-8
1. Beauty, Personal. I. Stone, Jeff
II. Gross, Kim Johnson. III. Newman, Judith. IV. Title: Chic Simple: Body.
V. Series.
RA778.N53   1994
646.7'2—dc20
94-15626
CIP

Manufactured in the United States of America
First Edition

To my mother, Evelyn Johnson, whose amazing attitude
toward life seems to defy aging; to the memory of
my father, Glenn Johnson, to whom my children and I
owe our long, lean limbs; and to my husband, David,
for one of life's more important ingredients—good loving.
K.J.G.

To my father, to whom I owe my tummy, and
my mother, to whom I owe my mustache.
J.S.

To Mr. Helpful. Thank you for services rendered.
J.N.

"The more you know, the less you need."

AUSTRALIAN ABORIGINAL SAYING

CONTENTS

USE US—PLEASE. After giving an overview of the body-mind connection, and explaining briefly the mechanics of the human animal, we've dissected (you'll pardon the expression) the body into discrete sections: **FACE, HAIR, SKIN, TORSO,** and **LIMBS.** Then we continue to subdivide: the chapter on the **FACE,** for example, consists of pages on the eyes, nose, mouth, lips, ears, etc. In our chapter "**WHOLENESS**" we give you our RX for maintaining a balance of mental and physical well-being. Under our explanation of each part of the body, we include a section called "MAINTENANCE": here, you'll find the latest information on what you need to do to keep that part of the body in optimal condition (for health and/or appearance). [VOICES] interspersed throughout the book, explain the gestalt of some of the most notable individuals working in the health, fitness, and medical fields today. In the back of the book we've included a section called " [🖼 *first aid*] ," where you'll find more body facts and beauty solutions. Take what's useful to you—and laugh at what's not. We're not interested in being Health-and-Beauty Police—but we want you to be aware of your options.

BODY

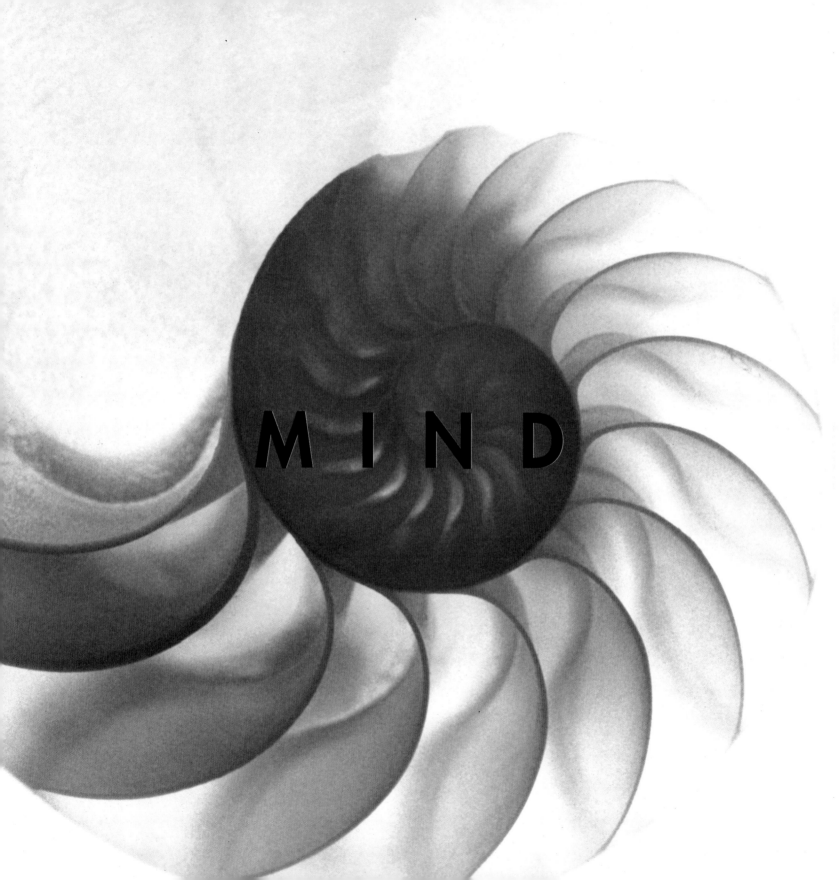

MIND

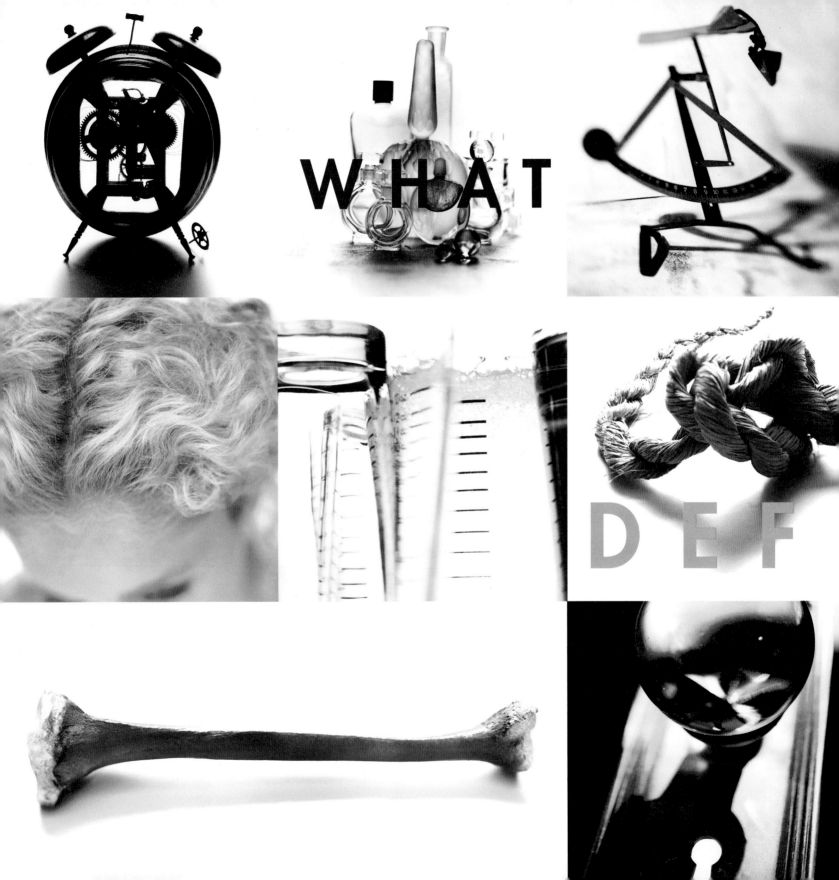

WHAT

DEF

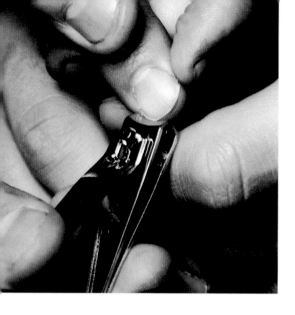

ME

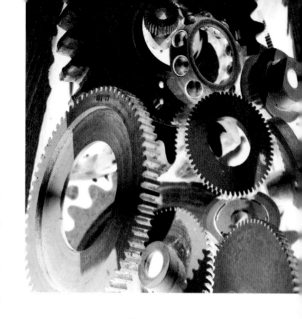

What is this amalgam of water, muscle, fat, and bone we live in? Is our body our essence, our Self, or is it merely a carapace we lug around, like a hermit crab its shell? This debate—just what exactly is the human body?—has occupied philosophers for centuries. This question is best left to them—but we hope this book will encourage you to consider the intricate relationship of the body and the mind. Because caring for one means caring for the other. CHIC SIMPLE BODY is about genuine self-help, the kind where you assume responsibility for your own health and contentment.

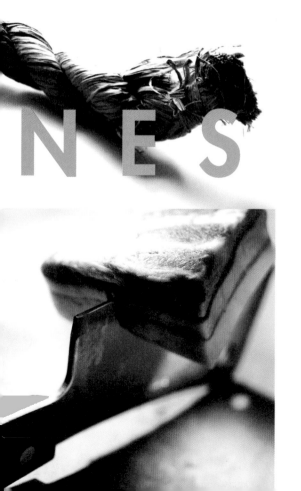

N E S

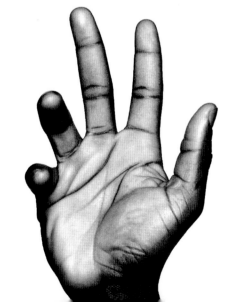

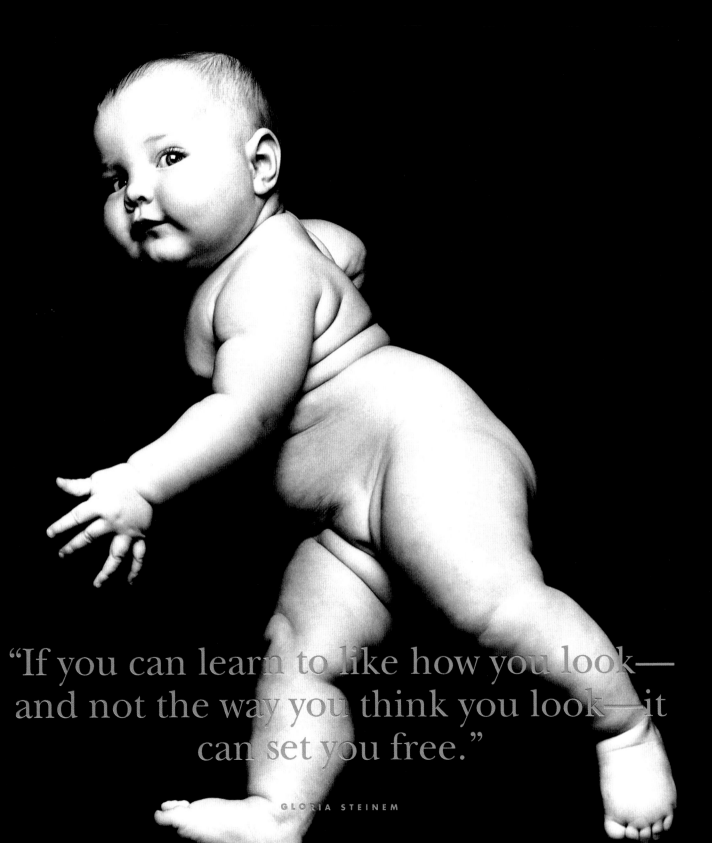

"If you can learn to like how you look—
and not the way you think you look—it
can set you free."

GLORIA STEINEM

B O D Y

ECTOMORPH, ENDOMORPH, MESOMORPH: WE LEARNED THESE TERMS IN JUNIOR HIGH, AND WE WORRIED ABOUT WHERE WE FIT IN. THE ectos (naturally scrawny) and endos (naturally plump) sat in the back of the class, plotting future revenge against the Mesos (the natural football players and cheerleaders). Since no one would go out with us anyway, our grades were higher and someday, we reasoned, we would return to our 10th high school reunions with better jobs and perfectly toned bodies. (Well, at least with better jobs.) We would triumph over genetics. A few of us actually did. In fact, body shape does influence more than our chance of getting a date on Saturday night. Apple-shaped men and women, whose fat is concentrated around the belly, are more prone to heart disease than "pears," whose fat coalesces around hips and thighs. A study at Duke University showed that women with apple shapes are at a higher risk for uterine cancer, and three times more likely to develop breast cancer. Research also shows that apple-shaped women who lose as little as 12 pounds can cut their risk of breast cancer almost in half. Why? Since fat cells surrounding the gut are larger and more metabolically active than those in buttocks, abdominal fat can have a profound impact on a myriad of chemical reactions, altering the blood levels of everything from cholesterol to glucose and sex hormones. Here's the good news: apple shapes have the advantage in weight loss, since it's easier to lose weight from the stomach than the hips.

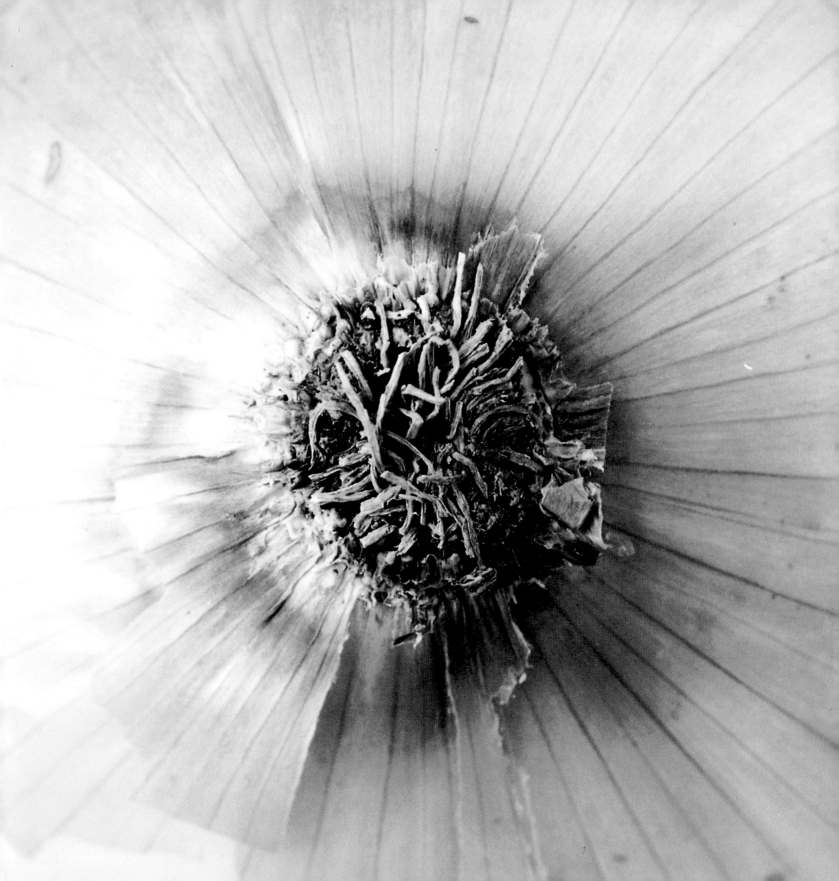

M I N D

THERE IS A MOMENT IN EVERY BABY'S LIFE WHEN HE LOOKS AT HIMSELF AND RECOGNIZES THE point where he ends and the rest of the world begins. It is this recognition of containment, of boundaries ("I can control the actions of my own body, but I can't levitate that Teddy bear over there"), that is the first acknowledgment of the Self. Later, we began to learn about what the mind can and cannot control—and the more we learn, the more ignorant we realize we are. Does that Uri Geller guy really bend those spoons through his mind? Can my friends on the Psychic Network predict my future—and if so, do I want to hear it? And what about people who speak in tongues or believe they're possessed by demons (maybe I could have levitated that Teddy bear after all)? What we *do* know is the mind has more power over health and well-being than we ever thought possible. Our mental outlook can revive or destroy us. If, as the saying goes, a mind is a terrible thing to waste, then the converse must be true: it's a wonderful thing to use.

"We know what we are, but know not what we may be."

WILLIAM SHAKESPEARE

An astonishing and best-selling proposition: Deepak Chopra, the author of *Perfect Health* and *Quantum Healing,* suggests that we can radically lengthen our lives (to 120 years or more) by altering our inner perspectives. Chopra maintains that his

DEEPAK CHOPRA, M.D.

iconoclastic theories are the biological corollaries to both quantum mechanics and Einstein's theory of relativity, namely, that there is no objective world independent of the observer and that time is a subjective force and therefore controllable subjectively. He cites numerous studies of the very old: what fortuitous combination of factors (from genetics to diet to capacity for joy) blessed them? Chopra proposes strategies for formulating healthy internal goals, freeing oneself from time pressure, staying in the present moment, and learning to be altruistic. Even those of us steeped in Western tradition can profoundly benefit from some Eastern attitude adjustment.

."Because the mind influences every cell in the body, human aging is fluid and changeable... Hundreds of research findings from the last three decades have verified that aging is much more dependent on the individual than was ever dreamed of in the past."

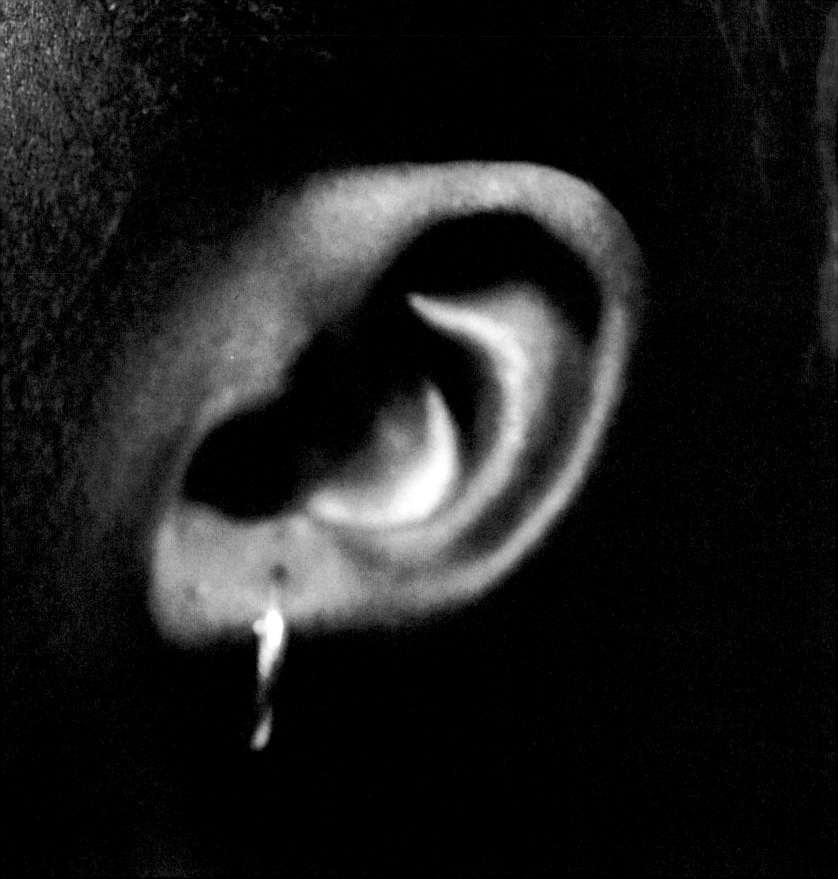

OPTIONS

FROM HAIRCUTS TO FACELIFTS, FROM CONTROL-TOP PANTY HOSE TO LIPOSUCTION, THE yearning for change is the one constant. Everyone wants to improve on what they are. Is there any part of the body that has not, at one time or another, been enhanced through artifice? Some ancient cultures thought fit to adorn body parts we've long ignored; aristocratic Egyptian women, for example, would outline the veins on their breasts with a bright blue plant dye before a rendezvous with their swains. Women seemed to have a higher tolerance for inconvenience, if not downright pain. In Ethiopian cultures, while women were stretching their necks with soldered-on neck rings, men restricted their ornamentation to body painting or molding clay in their hair. Today, women are even catching up to men in the one area of painful vanity once deemed "masculine"—namely, tattooing. "Beauty is truth, truth beauty," Keats proclaimed. Yet so much of what creates physical beauty in our culture involves, for both men and women, bending the truth a little.

"Maybe the less pain women inflict on their bodies, the more beautiful our bodies will look to us."

NAOMI WOLF

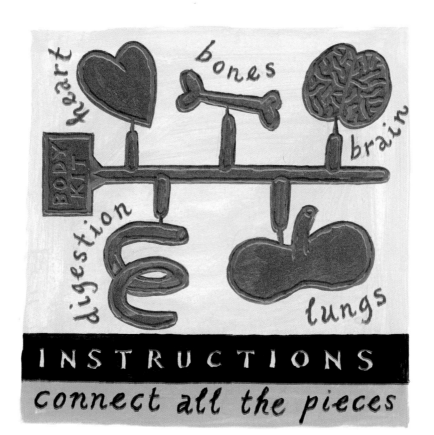

FRAMEWORK

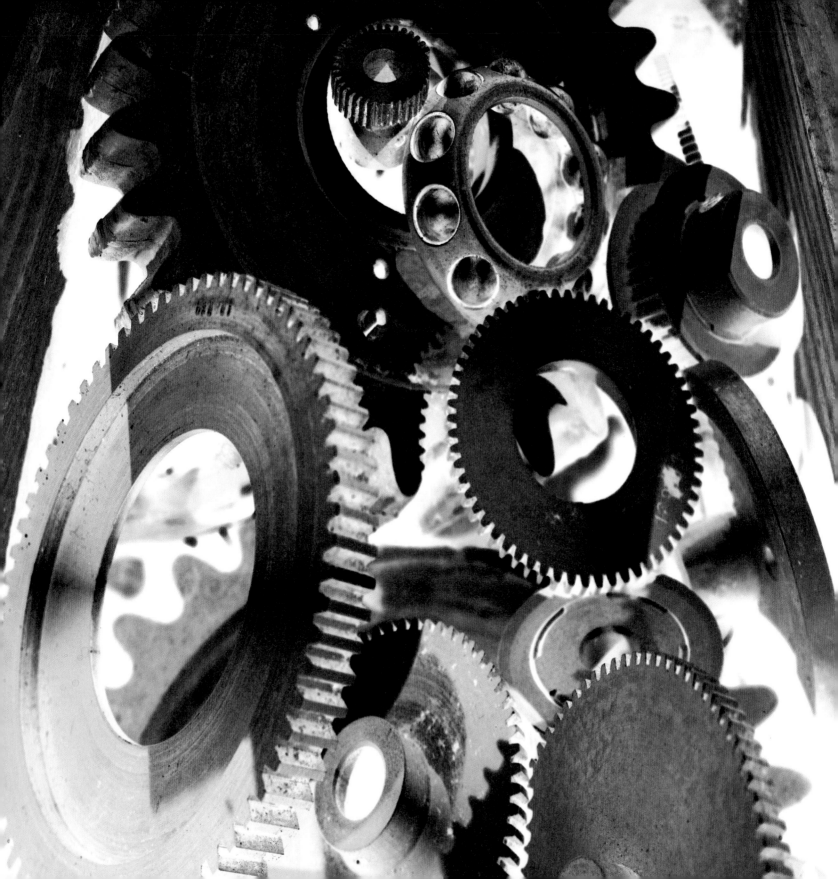

"The knee bone's connected to the thigh bone, and the thigh bone's connected to the hip bone..." The spirit that fueled that infectious little ditty was neatly contained in its final joyous refrain: "Now hear the word of the Lord." The song told us how every part of our body was interrelated, each part depending on others to function. And so we think of our bodies today. Consider the muscleman in the gym, all bulging muscles and testosterone; but with all the time he's spent building

WHAT MAKES ME WORK

bulk with anaerobic exercise, he may not have a high enough level of aerobic fitness to sprint up a flight of stairs. Or consider the 7-day-a-week exercise fanatic— aerobically fit, but so worried about gaining weight or otherwise "losing control" that she'd rather jeopardize her health than miss a workout. Every decision we make about our bodies has consequences. The secret is to strive for balance, where mind and body are enmeshed.

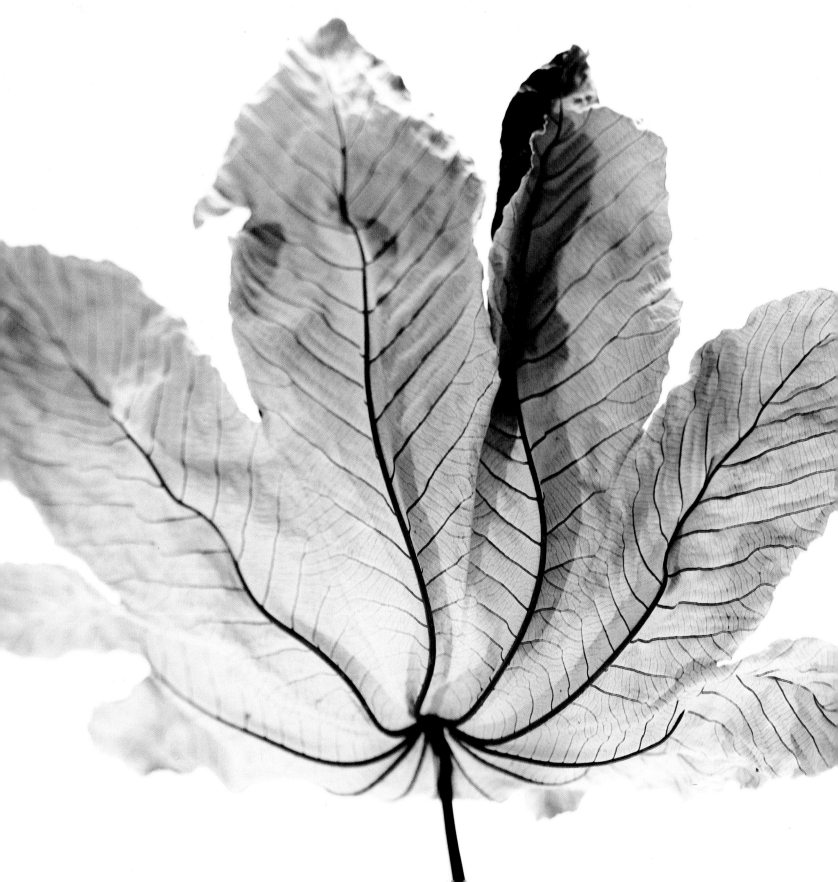

H E A R T

2,755,720,800. THAT'S THE NUMBER OF TIMES, IN AN AVERAGE LIFESPAN, THE HEART PUMPS BLOOD AROUND THE BODY. No wonder engineers have modeled pumps on this compact (8–10 ounces) piece of machinery. Yet this most mechanical of body parts is also considered the seat of human emotion. How did the heart come to symbolize love, fear, jealousy, compassion? Perhaps it's because it's the organ we're most aware of when our feelings shift. With fear, our hearts speed up; with sorrow, there's a sense of tightening; and with a loss of love—isn't there a feeling that something inside is broken?

BETTERING THE ODDS

50–70% lower risk, within 5 years of quitting, for former smokers compared with current smokers.

Regular moderate exercise

45% lower risk. Studies show endurance exercise increases the size of the coronary arteries.

Maintaining ideal weight

35–55% lower risk. Compared with people who are 20% or more above their ideal weight.

Consuming 1-2 glasses of alcoholic beverage per day

25–45% lower risk. Thought to lower chances of heart attack.

Taking one half an aspirin a day

33% lower risk. Aspirin has a mild anti-clotting factor, and it may lessen the chance of a stroke. Warning: This is not for everybody. Check with your doctor.

MAINTENANCE: A heart attack is quite simply the smothering of the heart that occurs when clogged arteries prevent it from getting enough blood. One in five men will die of a heart attack—which is why, until recently, heart disease was thought to be primarily a male thing, right up there with channel-surfing and the inability to ask for directions. In fact, heart disease is the second leading killer of U.S. women over the age of 40, second only to cancer; by age 55, heart disease is the leader. While women tend to suffer heart attacks at a later age than men, they die more frequently from the first heart attack, or are more likely to suffer second ones—possibly because early symptoms are sometimes misread by doctors who in the past have labeled the women merely "high-strung." As stated, there are physical courses of action one can take to better the odds. But more and more research has also shown that what and how you think about yourself and others can be just as significant in maintaining your heart.

[HEART *first aid—pages 193–94*]

"Changing behavior
for real healing to
address what under
not sufficient simply
like diet and exer
behaviors are only
self-perceptions. We
those perceptions
can lead to the

DR. DEAN ORNISH

Dr. Dean Ornish's Program for Reversing Heart Disease says it all: this time out, Ornish outlines his program for actually turning around serious heart problems without drugs or surgery, a program that also serves as a promoter of health and

is not always enough
occur. We need to
lies the behavior.. It's
to change behaviors
cise,. because our
manifestations of our
need also to change
of isolation that
set behaviors."

longevity. To the by now familiar insistence on a low-fat—preferably vegetarian—diet, moderate exercise, and stress management through meditation and yoga, Ornish adds a new mind-body injunction: love. Ornish believes, and his research studies tend to bear out, that increasing intimacy with others and communing with a "higher power" will, literally and figuratively, heal your heart.

"A cigarette is the perfect type of a perfect pleasure. It is exquisite and it leaves one unsatisfied."

OSCAR WILDE

L U N G S

FROM AN EARLY AGE, SMART LITTLE CHILDREN LEARN THE BENEFITS OF BEING ABLE TO HOLD THEIR BREATH—YOU TURN a lovely shade of blue and scare the bejesus out of your parents. (Later, you swear to the public you didn't inhale, and scare the bejesus out of your political handlers.) 10,000 to 12,000 quarts of air a day pass through our lungs. Lung power is will power; it reflects strength, good fortune, and vitality. We applaud the man who can blow out all the candles on his 50th birthday, because he's the one who'll outlive the rest of us.

CIGARETTE CHEMICALS

Nicotine

makes blood vessels constrict, cuts down the flow of blood and oxygen through your body, forcing your heart to pump faster.

Tar

damages delicate lung tissues. When the billions of tiny particles in cigarette smoke cook inside your lungs, some form a dark, sticky mass, containing chemicals that produce cancer in tests with animals.

Carbon monoxide

siphons oxygen out of red blood cells.

Dope dope

Marijuana is not "better" for the lungs than cigarettes; it is, in fact, considerably worse, as it contains far more foreign chemicals.

MAINTENANCE: During the aging process, we naturally lose lung tissue just as we lose muscle mass. However, we can stem the loss. **SMOKING:** It constricts the air passages and fills them with mucus; the air sacs inside the lungs disintegrate and lung muscles lose their elasticity, thereby the capacity to deliver oxygen into the bloodstream. **SECONDHAND SMOKE:** It has higher concentrations of some toxins than the smoke a smoker inhales. Statistically, non-smoking spouses of smokers have a significantly higher incidence of lung cancer than non-smoking spouses of non-smokers; and babies have a bigger incidence of respiratory illness in a home where one or both parents smoke. **TESTING:** After 40, get your lungs tested as regularly as your blood pressure. A quick test: take a deep breath, and then empty your lungs as quickly as you can. If it takes longer than 3 seconds to empty them completely, time to see a doctor.

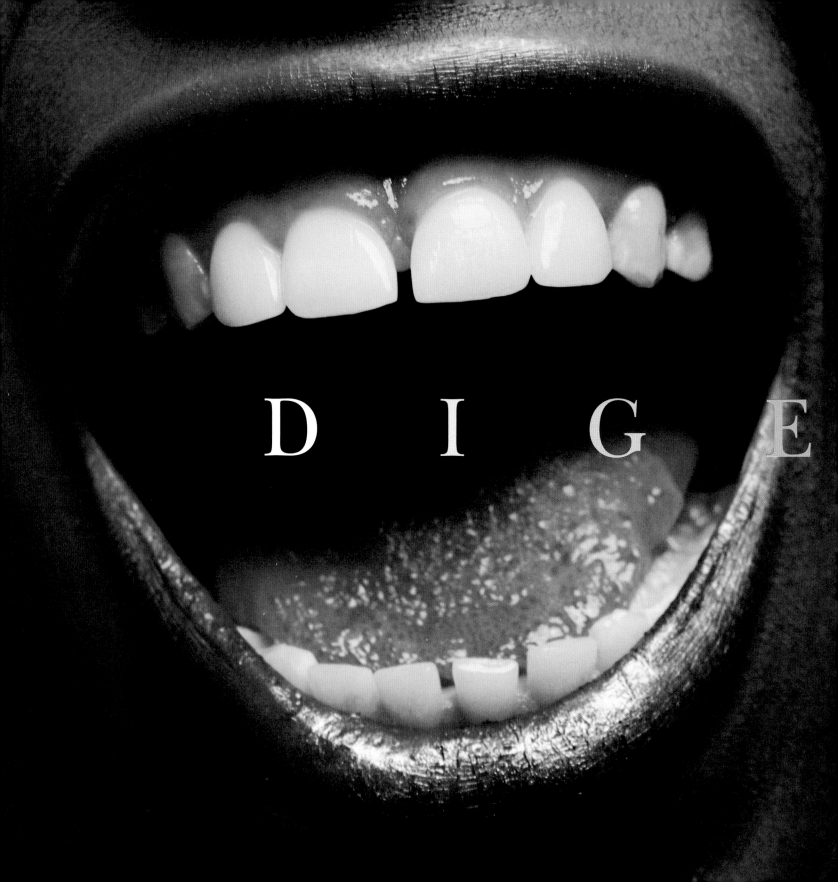

IF WE DIDN'T HAVE FOOD, WOULD WE HAVE FAMILIES? AS INFANTS, WE FIRST LEARN COMFORT AND TRUST THROUGH THE PERSON WHO FEEDS US; LATER, AT THE DINNER TABLE, WE LEARN THE ART OF CONVERSATION. TRY TO IMAGINE A FAMILY GET-TOGETHER THAT DOESN'T INVOLVE EATING, SINCE eating has created some of our most complex and subtle societal rituals. We can analyze family hierarchy by knowing who gets the Thanksgiving turkey drumstick and the largest piece of pie, and we know something about a person's social status if she knows where to place the fish fork. Paradoxically, food, our most primitive need, civilizes us.

S T I V E

MAINTENANCE: While some of us exist happily on a diet of nachos and jalapeños, others find anything stronger than Cream of Wheat unsettling. **AVOIDING HEARTBURN:** That painful burning sensation occurs when the lower esophageal sphincter, the valve at the junction of the esophagus and the stomach, is not properly closed, allowing the highly acidic contents of the stomach to back up into the esophagus. If you're prone to heartburn, avoid certain foods known to cause it: tomato products, citrus fruits and juices, coffee, fried/fatty foods—and, strangely, chocolate and peppermint. Cigarette smoking may also contribute.

FIGHTING FLATULENCE: Even the Queen of England does it: experts estimate that the average person passes gas about 14 times a day. Intestinal gas is a normal by-product of digestion. Unfortunately, some of the healthiest foods—high-fiber carbohydrates like beans and cruciferous vegetables—are also those that produce the most gas (another reason to live on Twinkies). A new product on the market, Beano, contains an enzyme that helps break down certain indigestible carbohydrates. **AVOIDING ULCERS:** Contrary to popular opinion, stress does not cause ulcers. Nor does coffee or spicy food. There's increasing evidence that ulcers are caused by a type of bacteria.

[DIGESTIVE *first aid—page 194*]

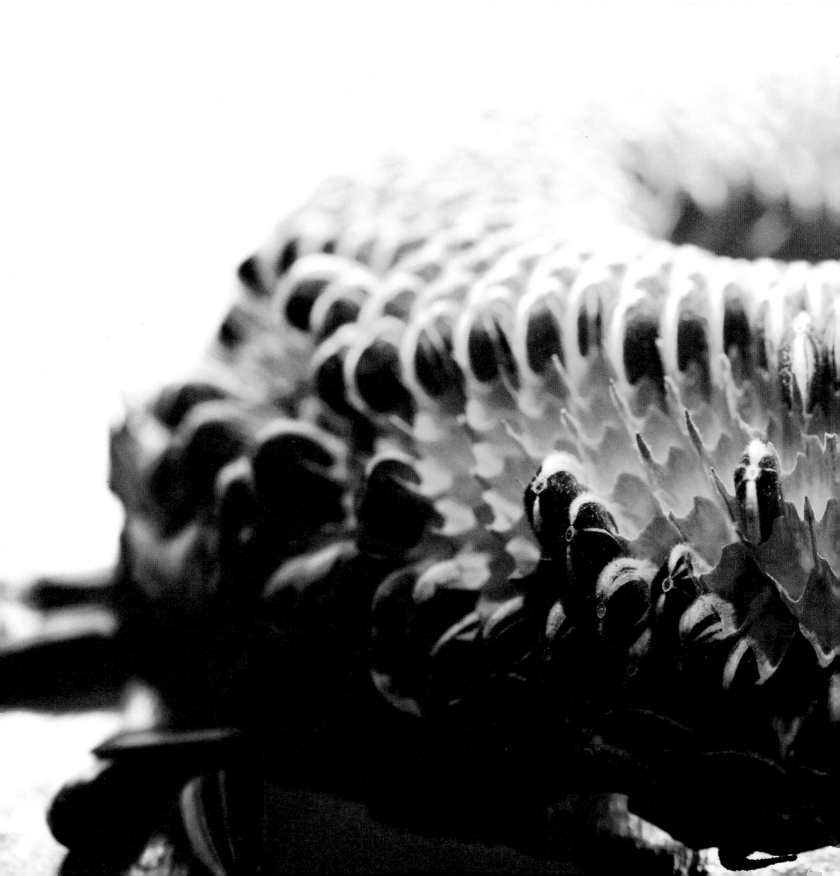

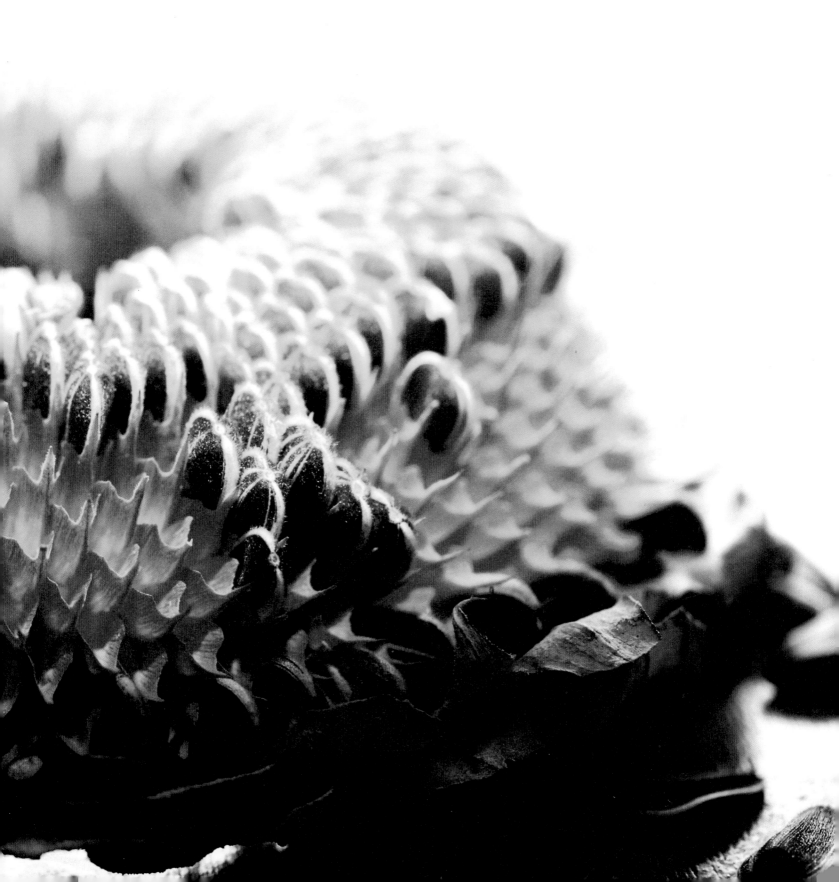

B O N E S

WHY IS THE UNIVERSAL SIGN FOR "DEATH" OR "POISON" A SKULL AND CROSSBONES? WHY DO WE GROW UP BEING FRIGHTENED OF A DANCING SKELETON AT HALLOWEEN AND NOT, SAY, A DANCING GALLBLADDER? PERHAPS BECAUSE, LONG AFTER WE'RE DEAD, THE SKELETON IS THE LAST PART OF US THAT'S recognizably human. Bones are a reminder of mortality, more so than our not-so-solid flesh, which melts quickly. Just as "the bones" of a project are its fundamental plan, so the bones of a human being—the dense, rigid, porous connective tissue—reveal the essence of the human design.

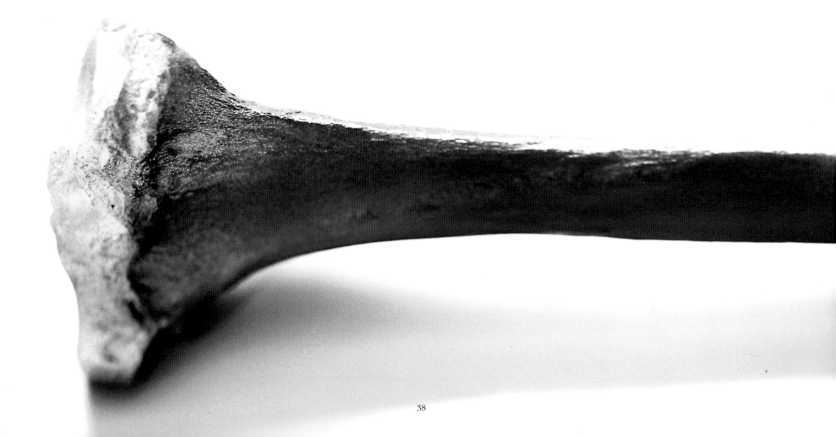

MAINTENANCE: The most common (and largely preventable) bone problem facing Americans today is osteoporosis, "porous bones"—a potentially crippling condition characterized by dramatic bone loss through the skeletal system. Nearly one third of all women over the age of 65 have some degree of osteoporosis. The result? Shrinkage and "dowager's hump"—from a compressed vertebrae column—and bones that can be broken by a minor fall or a major hug. Caucasian and Asian women are more at risk than African-Americans. Women have osteoporosis

Where to find calcium?

- Vitamin D–enriched low-fat milk, which helps the body absorb calcium.
- Fruits and cabbage-family vegetables that contain boron and vitamin K, which help the body retain calcium.
- Vitamin supplements, preferably calcium carbonate. Do not become vitamin-happy; more than the RDA for calcium can interfere with the absorption of other necessary minerals and increase the risk of kidney stones.

at a rate 8 times higher than men for several reasons. **MENOPAUSE:** After menopause, women are less able to absorb that crucial osteoporosis preventative, calcium, in their diets. **PREGNANCY:** Pregnancy and lactation draw heavily on a woman's calcium resources. **DIET:** Women tend to diet more frequently than men, and have greater fluctuations in weight. The result: prolonged periods of nutrient depletion. The key to avoiding osteoporosis in later years is stockpiling calcium in the body when you're best able to absorb it—in the years before menopause.

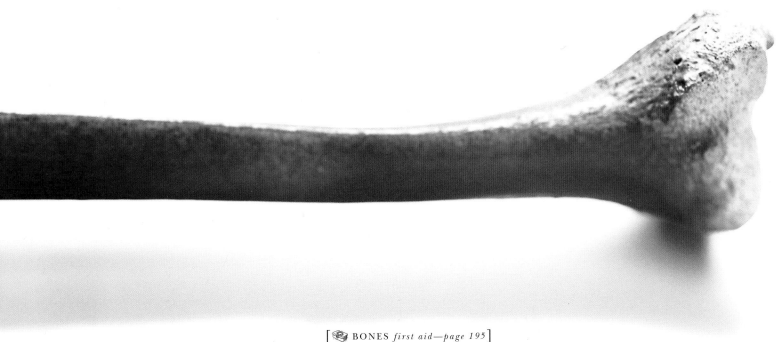

[BONES *first aid—page 195*]

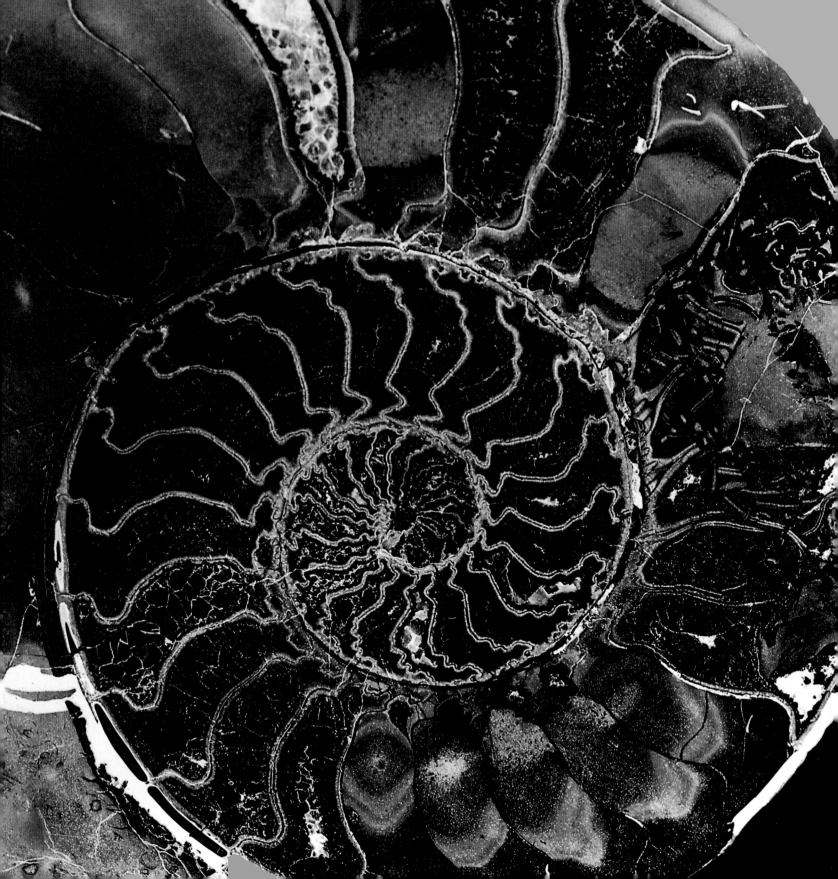

B R A I N

WE KNOW THAT EACH SIDE OF THE BRAIN CONTROLS THE OPPOSITE SIDE OF THE BODY, AND THAT THE RIGHT BRAIN HEMISPHERE IS associated with musical perception, visual patterns, and emotion, while the left hemisphere is associated with verbal skills. But for every leap in understanding of brain function, there are more profound mysteries: how do we acquire language? What's the secret of a "photographic" memory? When a patient receives a brain injury, how does one side of the brain take over the functions of the damaged side (as frequently happens)? How can so-called idiots savants be so profoundly damaged, yet have one extraordinary skill? The brain has been as reluctant to give up its secrets as the body.

MAINTENANCE: Scientists estimate we use only a small fraction of the brain power allotted to us. (Does this mean, if we used a teeny bit more the world would never have known about Beavis and Butt-head?) **IMPROVING MEMORY:** One of the great terrors of aging is the fear we'll lose our memories; in fact, the brain is one of the few organs of the body that degenerates very minimally with age. Unless memory loss has organic causes—as is the case in Alzheimer's disease—the secret to maintaining mental acuity is, simply, mental activity: just as with the body, it's a case of "Use it or lose it." Read. Listen to music. Watch "Jeopardy" every day. Be a participant, not a spectator. **MIGRAINES:** Migraines (from a Greek root meaning "half a head") typically involve an intense, throbbing pain on one side of the head. While no one knows exactly what causes migraines, it's now suspected that the neurotransmitter serotonin may have something to do with them. Serotonin levels in the blood drop during migraine attacks, causing vessels in the head to spasm painfully. Estrogen has a direct influence on serotonin levels, which may be why many women sufferers tend to have migraines around their periods.

[BRAIN *first aid—page 195*]

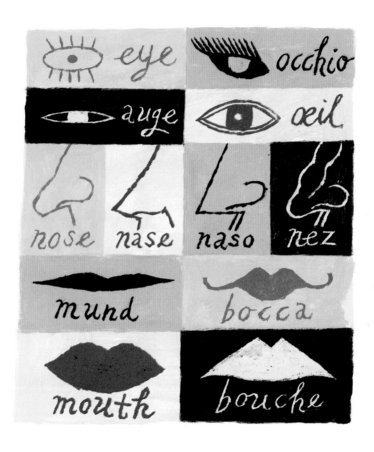

FACE

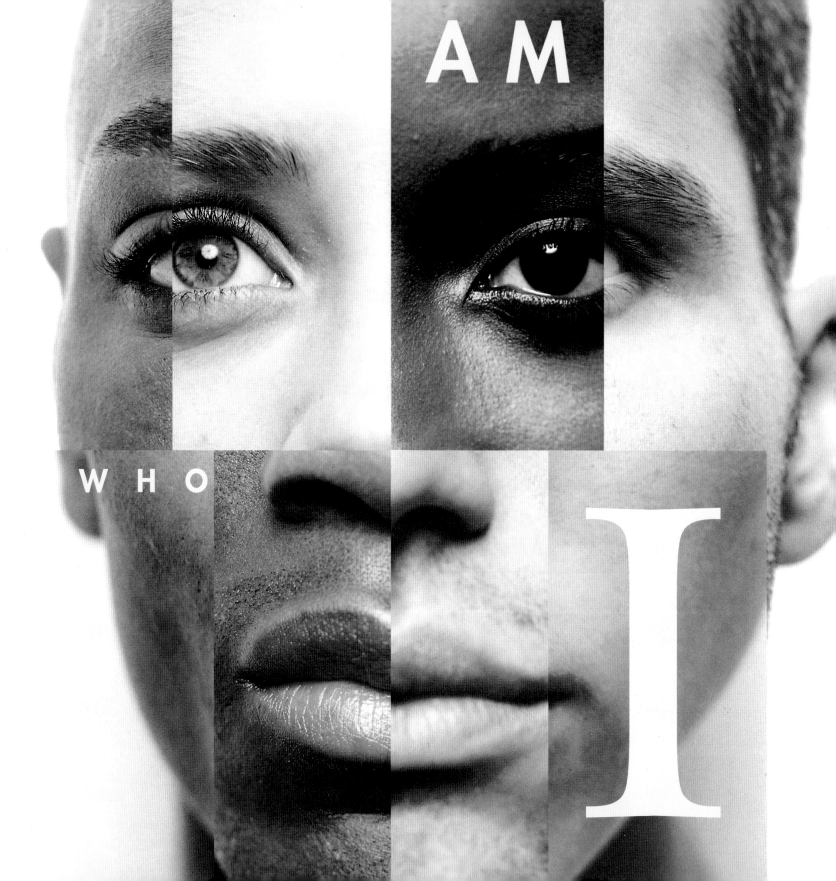

It begins in our childhood, when fairy-tale heroes are tall and handsome, heroines are fair, and evildoers are old and ugly. The Gorgon's hideousness turned men to stone; Helen of Troy's beauty inspired men to war. The power of the face continues throughout our lives. Studies prove that attractive men and women are more likely to reap life's rewards: they're cuddled more as infants, do better in school, and are rewarded with higher pay and better jobs. Traditionally, a woman's beauty has allowed her to make leaps in wealth and social status: a woman's face can literally become her fortune. Men's faces have always reaped social and financial gain: what would Porfirio Rubirosa have been to Barbara Hutton and Doris Duke without those cheekbones? Happily, there are counterbalances to the tyranny of physiognomy, since perceptions of beauty change from era to era and culture to culture. Today's waif supermodel was yesterday's shunned consumptive. While America is still a society that worships willowy bodies and young faces, look around you: quirky bodies and older faces are assuming their rightful places among the beautiful.

FACIAL SKIN

PEEL AN APPLE AND WATCH IT BROWN. THAT, SCIENTISTS SPECULATE, IS WHAT HAPPENS IN THE HUMAN AGING PROCESS: LIKE the apple flesh exposed to air, human flesh is oxidizing. Sun exposure and pollutants generate oxidants known as free radicals—destructive molecules in the body that cause cell damage by stealing electrons from other body cells, destabilizing oxygen molecules, and weakening or killing cells in the process. While the antioxidant theory is still in its infancy, we do know for sure that sunlight and smoking are The Enemy.

The free radical/ antioxidant theory

Our bodies contain natural antioxidants that combine with free radicals, preventing them from damaging DNA and enzymes in the skin. As we age, there are fewer antioxidants in our system.

What it means

The free radicals, i.e., the bad guys, are the "rust" of the body. Bonding with the free radicals, antioxidants prevent the rust from beginning.

The antioxidants

The big three are beta-carotene, vitamin A, and vitamin E—they can be taken in supplements, or in green leafy vegetables like spinach or broccoli.

MAINTENANCE: **CHRONOLOGY OF THE SKIN:** In the TWENTIES the skin is lubed up with oil and acne; shiny patches are common. In your THIRTIES, as oiliness wanes, horizontal lines on the forehead generally make their debut . The FORTIES generally see the formation of vertical frown lines between the eyebrows, puffiness under the eyes, and slackening of skin underneath the neck. By the FIFTIES the nasolabial line—the crease running from the corners of the nose to the corners of the mouth—have deepened and extended down the jaw. Welcome to the beginning of jowls. As a layer of subcutaneous fat melts away in the SIXTIES, wrinkles become more noticeable. Pinched skin doesn't snap back into place. **AVOID:** Smoking, rapid weight loss (skin loses elasticity), lack of exercise, and, most of all, sun.

"Being natural is simply a pose, and the most irritating pose I know of."

OSCAR WILDE

[FACIAL SKIN *first aid—pages 195–97*]

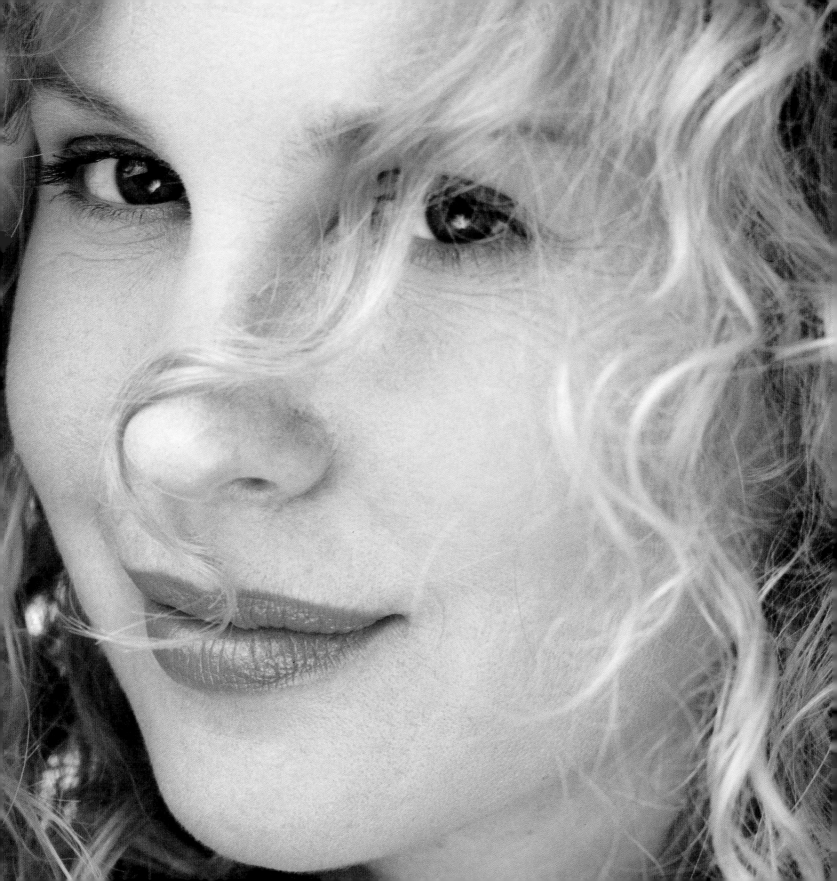

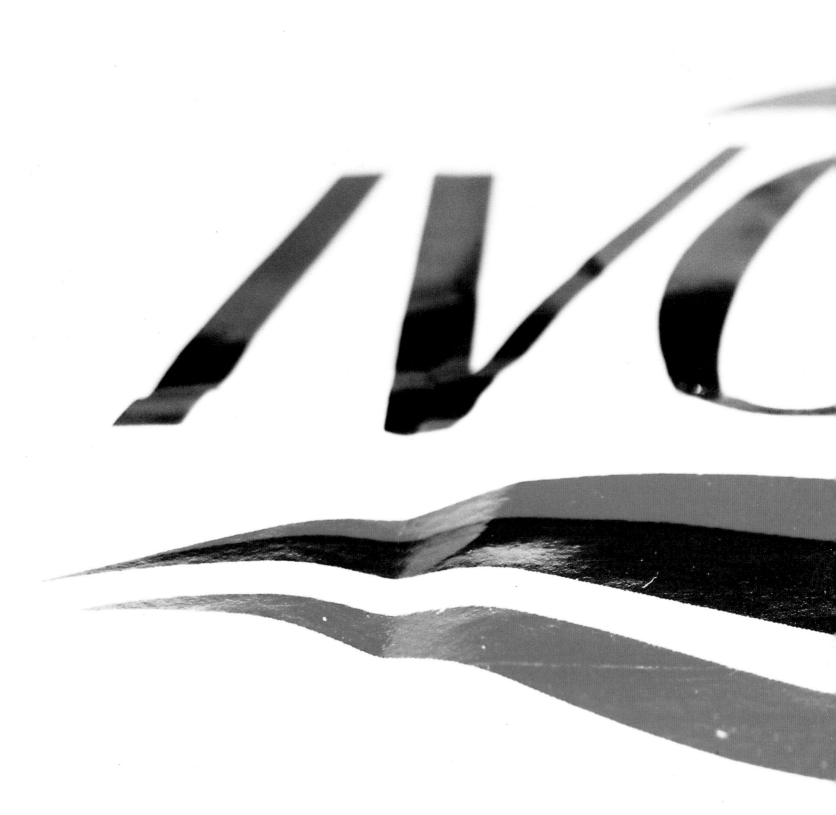

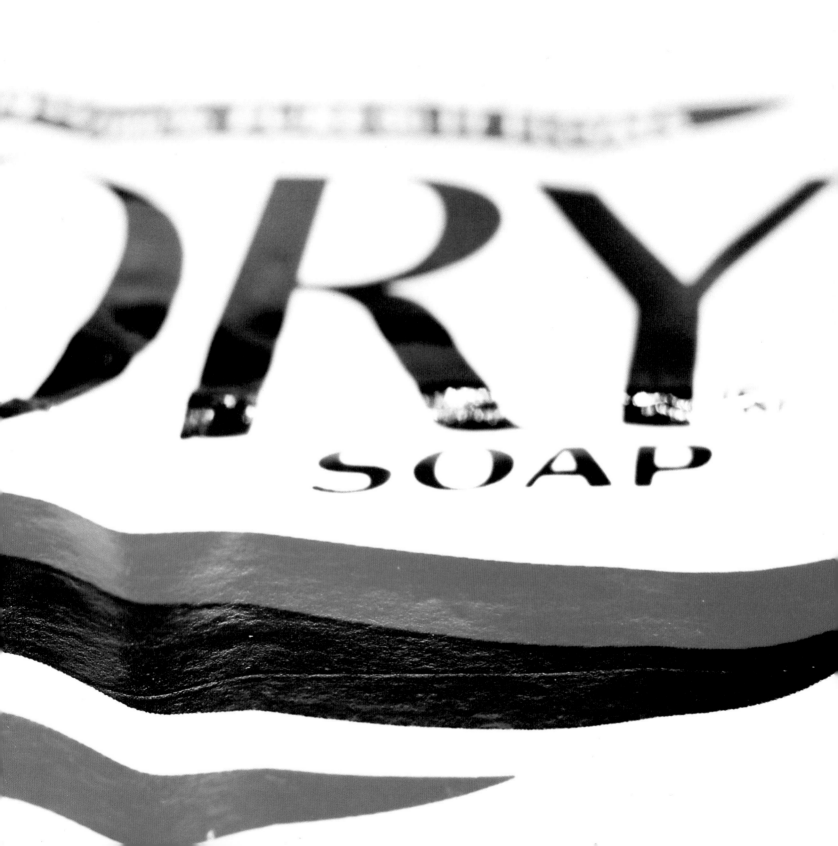

Cleansing and M

HOW TO WASH YOUR FACE: A cleanser, followed by water; the washcloth is optional. That's it. If your skin is oily, washing frequently or with too much enthusiasm is a mistake: the sebaceous glands, which secrete skin oils, go into overdrive when oil is vigorously scrubbed away, thereby increasing oil production. Look for products with witch hazel, which makes skin feel fresh without drying it out. If skin is dry, think cleansing bars, not soap. Some soaps contain detergent, which leeches water out of the skin. Think pure. **WATER, WATER, EVERYWHERE:** Ever wonder why people in very humid climates have skin that seems to age more slowly than those in dry climates? Their skin is thoroughly saturated with water, which makes it appear moist and supple. Researchers speculate that water keeps the lipids, or fat molecules, in the skin loose and flexible; lack of water makes the lipids rigid, which causes skin to look dry. Since we can't all move to a rain forest, we've got to do the next best thing: keep skin clean yet saturated with moisture. **MOISTURIZING FROM WITHIN:** Don't wait until you're thirsty to drink fluids, because by the time you're thirsty, you've already been dehydrated for quite a while. Try to drink eight 8-ounce glasses of non-caffeinated liquid a day (caffeine products and

Moisturizing

alcohol causes dehydration by putting the kidneys into overdrive). **MOISTURIZING FROM WITHOUT:** Soaking yourself in a tub for twenty minutes, and then lathering on a layer of heavy-duty moisturizer. **THE MOISTURIZER MYTH:** Cosmetics companies would like us to believe that moisturizers seep into our skin and plump them up with liquid. In fact, moisturizers do not penetrate the epidermis, the skin's outer layer, at all. The best they can do is act as humectants, helping water cling, limpetlike, to the skin's surface. The very best humectants are the cheapest, and also the messiest and most impractical to use—think about spending a day covered in Vaseline, and you get the picture. (If you can stand the ick factor, though, try petroleum jelly or even vegetable oil at night—on clean skin, covered up to protect the bedclothes.) More expensive (and aesthetically pleasing) lotions and emollients contain more water than oil, and need to be reapplied more frequently. **SMOKE:** About 467,000 tons of tobacco are burned indoors each year. Smoke releases a laundry list of toxins that impair blood circulation and inhibit the skin's ability to cleanse itself through natural sloughing. It damages not only your skin but the skin of people around you. Even the dog will thank you.

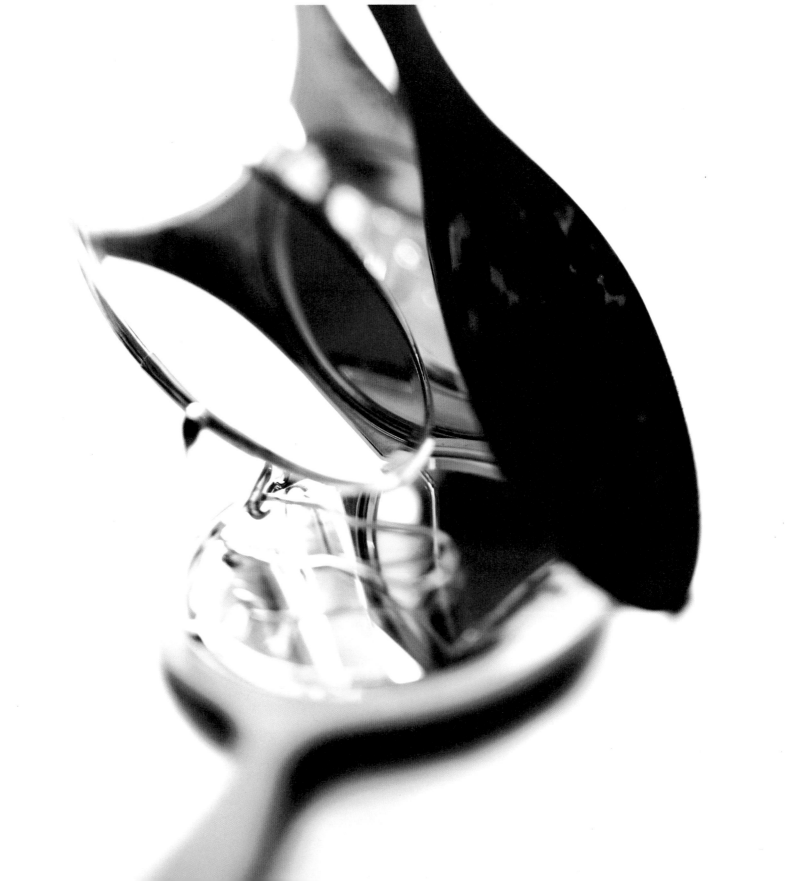

BEAUTY

WOULD YOU DIE FOR BEAUTY? WOMEN THROUGHOUT THE CENTURIES HAVE—OR AT LEAST SUFFERED MIGHTILY FOR IT. IN EARLY ROME, STERILITY AND STILL-births from lead poisoning were common-place, thanks in part to the white lead used for women's face powder. Early lipsticks contained dangerous metals such as lead and mercury, which went right into the bloodstream. During the Italian Renaissance and later in Victorian England, women happily put drops of belladonna—a poisonous plant in the nightshade family—into their eyes to enlarge their pupils before an evening's entertainment. Never mind that belladonna rendered them so sensitive to light as to almost blind them; the drug mimicked the eye dilation of sexual arousal. During the 18th century, women were willing to eat Arsenic Complexion Wafers, which destroyed the hemoglobin in the blood, to give them that alabaster, opalescent hue. In 17th-century Romania, a countess slaughtered peasant virgins so that she could bathe in their blood and stay youthful. Come to think of it, how does a vampire retain his youthful charms? It's all in that plasma. And you thought leg waxing was bad.

> "I require only three things of a man. He must be handsome, ruthless, and stupid."
>
> DOROTHY PARKER

53

"The ideology of semi-starvation undoes feminism; what happens to women's bodies happens to our minds... The more financially independent, in control of events, educated, and sexually autonomous women become in the world, the more impoverished, out of control, foolish, and sexually insecure we are asked to feel in our bodies."

Naomi Wolf says of *The Beauty Myth,* "This is not a conspiracy theory, it doesn't have to be." Yet at times it sounds like one. Wolf maintains that pervasive media images of frighteningly thin young women as the female "ideal" were propagated when women

NAOMI WOLF

became a political threat to the status quo: namely, with the rebirth of feminism. One of her most compelling chapters—"Hunger"—cites the recent exponential rise in eating disorders and obsessive dieting in very young women while noting that "a generation ago, the average model weighed 8 percent less than the average American woman, whereas today she weighs 23 percent less." Wolf makes the case that even if women do achieve this "ideal," they will be in a state of semi-starvation, probably infertile, and without energy. If they don't, they will feel like failures. Conforming to society's ideals will harm us physically and mentally, but refusing to conform, at least to some extent, results in partial exile. The overall effect is to psychologically strip women of their power.

SIMPLE
MAKEUP
TEN STEPS
TEN MINUTES
(or less)

(or, How to apply makeup to look like you're not wearing makeup)
courtesy of renowned makeup artist Bobbi Brown

[MAKEUP *first aid—pages 197–99*]

1 Start with a foundation half a shade lighter than your skin tone. Pat it on blemishes and blend it around your eyes as a concealer. **2** Use a slightly darker foundation (one that matches your skin) around your nose and chin to even out skin tones. **3** Apply loose powder with a puff, not a brush; a puff provides overall coverage. Look for powder with a yellow undertone, because translucent powders tend to sap color from the skin. **4** To define eyebrows, brush them over with a brown matte eye shadow applied with a stiff, slanted brush. The lighter your hair, the lighter the shade of brown. **5** Define the lower lash line with a brown or black pencil. A key step: Retrace your eyeliner with a matching shade of eye shadow—the shadow will adhere to the liner, making it last longer. **6** Apply a medium-tone eye shadow over the entire lid. **7** Optional: Use an eyelash curler if eyelashes are very straight. **8** Apply two to three light coats of black mascara better than one heavy application. Blot to prevent clumping. **9** Apply blush to the apple of cheek. **10** Apply lipstick—but only to the bottom lip. Purse lips together and rub.

S I M

EYELINER SHARPENER:
Don't be tempted to sharpen
pencils with them, too, as this will
dull the blade.

EYELASH CURLER:
Compress eyelashes three times
for a 5-second count each time.

All you need to put your best face forward:

Eyeliner sharpener, eyelash curler,
tweezers, blush brush, eye shadow
applicator, lash and brow tool.

T O O L S

P L E

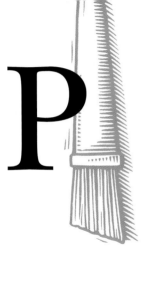

EYE SHADOW APPLICATOR:
Use one shadow applicator per color;
otherwise, will become muddy.

LASH AND BROW TOOL:
Brush keeps eyebrows groomed;
lash comb separates eyelashes after
application of (potentially goopy)
mascara.

TWEEZERS:
Hair today, gone…. Tweezers
with blunt-angled tips are preferable
for eyebrow maintenance (sharp,
needlelike tips are better for, say,
removing splinters).

BLUSH BRUSH:
Best: Big, fluffy brushes
that spread powder evenly over
cheeks—resulting in an all-over glow,
not a Bozo-like splotch of color.

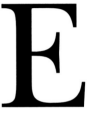

[MAKEUP TOOLS *first aid—page 199*]

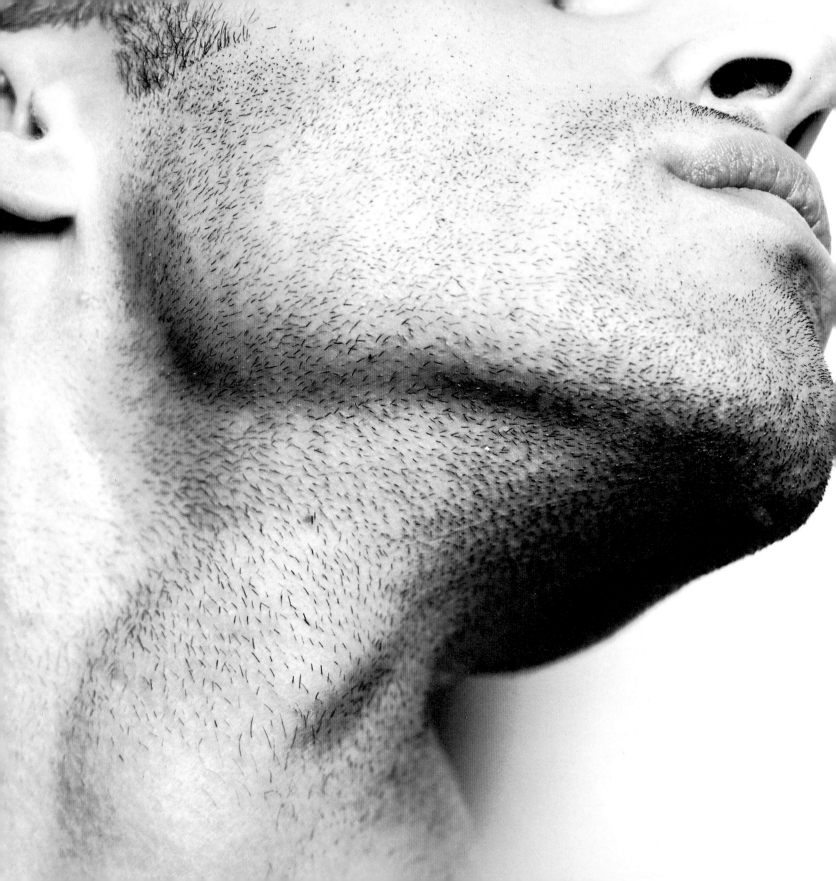

FACIAL HAIR

MEN. A man's beard and mustache appear at puberty, somewhere between 13 to 18, increase into the early 20s, then stabilize. Ear hair usually doesn't become apparent until a man hits his 40s or 50s. A gray beard usually—but not always—precedes a gray head. In some cultures beards remain *de rigueur*: Hasidic Jews and Amish men, for example, are prohibited from shaving their beards.

MAINTENANCE: **STUBBLE:** Less than 24 hours after you shave, a man's beard makes its appearance again, making you look either like Tom Selleck or that guy who hangs around OTB all day. Be forewarned: most men look like Mr. OTB with a couple of days' growth. **BEARD MAINTENANCE:** Those who do not want their beards to act as crumb catchers should keep them reasonably well trimmed; a barber can do it and there are electric shavers that have built-in guides. Don't use soap to wash your beard but shampoo it when you do your hair. **AVOIDING INGROWN HAIRS:** Most common in men with coarse, curly hair—especially African-American and Mediterranean men. Scrub lightly with a washcloth every day to keep pores clean and open.

WOMEN. The amount of facial hair is genetically determined, but it will fluctuate with changing hormone levels. Consequently, the Pill can cause an increase in facial hair growth. Also, older women tend to become hairier as the level of estrogen in the body falls in relation to testosterone levels.

MAINTENANCE: **BLEACHING** lightens hair on the face (really a bad idea if your skin happens to be dark). Chemical cream **DEPILATORIES** dissolve hair at the root but need to be used quite frequently and may irritate skin. **WAXING**—applying strips of wax to the hairy area and then ripping it off—works wonderfully, removing hair below root level. For those with sensitive skin, face waxing can cause skin to break out. **ELECTROLYSIS**—destruction of hair follicles by running a mild electric current through them—is the only permanent method of hair removal. It can be pricey, and often has to be repeated several times. **BAD HAIR SOLUTION:** Shaving. Does not make hair grow back faster or thicker, as reputed; however, it may irritate the skin. Plus, stubble on a woman is unlikely to have the same turn-on quotient as stubble on Tom Selleck.

[FACIAL HAIR *first aid—pages 199–201*]

"WRINKLES," AS ONE WAG OBSERVED, ARE "THE LONG-SERVICE STRIPES EARNED IN THE HARD CAMPAIGN OF LIFE." BUT DO WE NEED ALL OF OUR WRINKLES TO PROVE THAT WE'RE WISE? MEN AND WOMEN WITH THE MONEY, TIME, AND INCLINATION CAN DO SOMETHING ABOUT WRINKLES THESE days. Here's what's available in the United States (there are treatments in France that aren't yet available here including a wrinkle filler made of catgut), in ascending order of effectiveness:

ALPHA HYDROXY ACIDS (AHAs), the latest weapon in the wrinkle wars, are also effective against age spots and sun damage. Derived from fruits, plants, and sour milk, AHAs are exfoliants; they work by attaching to the dry, dead skin cells on the skin's surface and causing them to flake off when a facial mask is applied. ADVANTAGE: AHAs don't cause reddening, burning, or photosensitivity like Retin-A, Renova, or stronger chemical peels. They're also useful for pregnant women who often can't use Retin-A, since it's a vitamin A derivative and high amounts can cause birth defects; darker women find it causes lightening, darkening, or mottling of skin. DISADVANTAGE: Are they drugs or cosmetics? So far, the FDA is allowing AHAs to be sold in mild solutions by cosmetics companies over the counter, as long as companies don't claim on their packaging anything more than glowing, "revived" complexions. AHA potions in cosmetics range from 1.2 to 5 percent concentrations— but in treatments given by dermatologists, the acid content may go as high as 70 percent. **RETIN-A AND RENOVA:** Women have been dabbing themselves in Retin-A since 1988; Renova, its milder cousin, has just become available. Once used to fight teenage acne, both Renova and Retin-A are powerful exfoliants, sloughing off the dead cells that clutter the surface of aging skin and make it look dull. The ingredient in both is tretinoin, or all-trans-retinoic acid. (In laboratory animals, retinoids have been found to prevent skin, breast, bladder, and lung tumors.) ADVANTAGE: Here's the consensus of scientists: Retin-A and Renova do reverse sun damage—fine lines, leathery texture, and age spots. DISADVANTAGE: But both also increase the skin's photosensitivity. Renova may still be something of an improvement over Retin-A, because it's delivered to the skin in a moisturizing base, making it less irritating. **CHEMICAL PEELS:** These treatments are a serious business: performed in a doctor's office, they are extremely effective against wrinkling and hyperpigmentation. Problem is, the stronger the peel solution, the more the skin irritation and the longer the patient will be out of commission—sometimes over two weeks. **DERMABRASION:** Dermabrasion is like a chemical sandpapering of the skin, and is usually recommended only for deep acne scarring. **COLLAGEN, FAT INJECTIONS, AND—GORE-TEX? COLLAGEN** is a liquid protein that's extracted from cowhide and injected into the inner layers of skin, which fills in fine wrinkles and gives skin a plumper appearance. **ADVANTAGE:** The procedure takes no more than 15 minutes, and is relatively inexpensive. **DISADVANTAGE:** Unfortunately, the effects only last about six months, and there is ongoing controversy in the U.S. about possible connections between collagen and autoimmune diseases. **FAT INJECTIONS,** on the other hand, pose no problem as far as allergies or rejection go—the fat is taken from another site on the patient's anatomy, like the buttocks or thighs, and injected under the skin. But fat injections, which are considerably more expensive, don't actually fill in wrinkles. They can, however, temporarily fill in hollowed cheeks, make lips more pouty, and plump up bony hands. Newest wrinkle on the wrinkle-filling front: **POLYTETRAFLUOROETHYLENE,** a synthetic material patented by the people who brought us Gore-Tex. This soft, pliable material is being inserted into the nasolabial folds (frown lines) around the mouth, to "plump" up the lines and make them less noticeable. **BOTULISM INJECTIONS.** Okay, so it's a lethal bacteria. But scientists are eliminating the frown line that forms between the eyebrows by injecting tiny drops of botulism just beneath the skin. Wrinkles happen because skin is sticking to muscles that contract underneath it. If the muscle can't contract, you can't form a wrinkle. A drop of Botox actually paralyzes the muscles in the face that cause the frown line. The effects of paralysis only last a few months. **FACELIFTS:** Technology in facelifts is changing fast. A few years ago, a facelift was merely a matter of tightening skin over the face, and snipping away the excess—which can make a woman look like she's fighting her way through a wind tunnel. These days, fat and muscle underneath the facial skin are being removed and shifted around. The result (sometimes): a face which looks not merely tighter but…different. Sometimes really different.

Number of facelifts performed yearly in the U.S. by board-certified plastic surgeons
40,000
Ratio of female facelifts to male facelifts
about 7 to 1

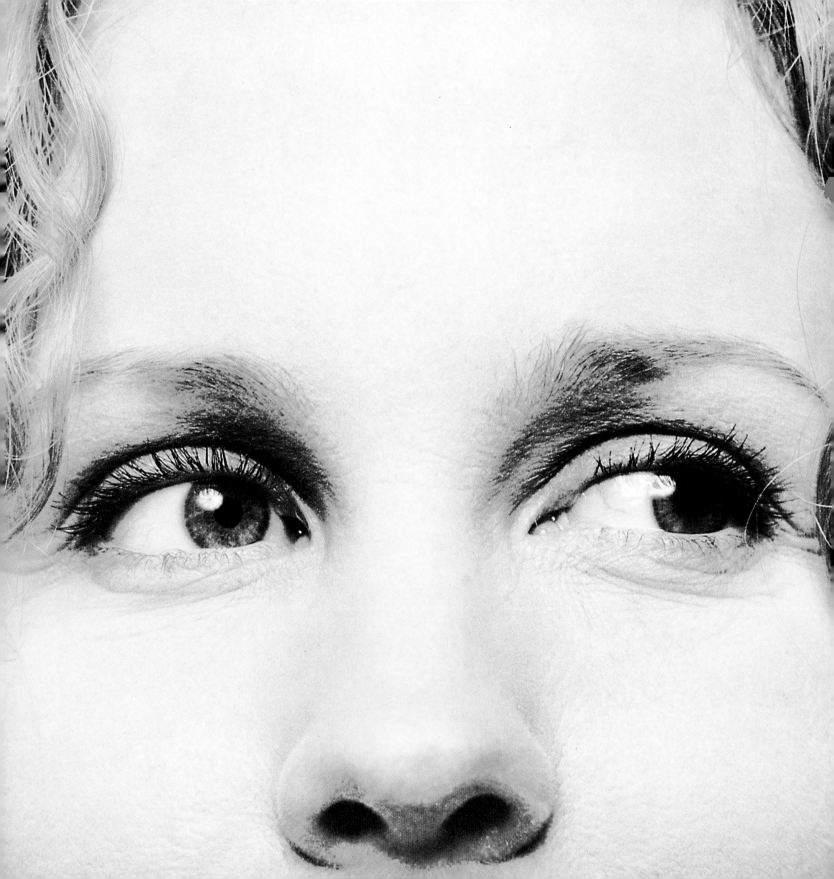

E Y E S

"THE EYES," RALPH WALDO EMERSON ONCE SAID, "INDICATE THE ANTIQUITY OF THE SOUL"— ALTHOUGH MOST OF US WOULD prefer that our souls appear not quite so ancient after an evening of margaritas. Eyes are the first feature we notice, and the last we forget. No other bodily reaction evokes human empathy faster than the shedding of tears. The majority of Americans will spend some part of their lives wearing corrective lenses. The gradual blurring of vision is, in a sense, a brilliant evolutionary adaptation. Why should the wrinkles that accumulate with time remain in clear, sharp focus? Nature, like a clever cameraman, puts its own discreet soothing gauze on the lens.

To reduce redness
Eye drops that promise to "get the red out" use naphazoline, a vasoconstrictor that shrinks the blood vessels artificially, temporarily blanching the white of the eye. Drops should be used only occasionally. If you find yourself using them daily, visit your doctor.

To reduce puffiness
Soak cotton balls in half ice water, half cold whole milk, and place one over each eye for 15 minutes. The icy temperature plus the fats in the whole milk have an anti-inflammatory effect.

To conceal dark circles
Circles are hereditary and not readily treatable by plastic surgery; they're caused by blood vessels being very close to the skin surface, lending a bluish cast. Put concealer all around the eyes—not just under them—and blend.

MAINTENANCE: Arguably, our eyes are our most expressive feature; the cumulative effect of smiles and frowns is etched into our facial topography. With all this movement, the thin, delicate skin around the eyes is the first area of the face to show aging. The first line of defense? A good pair of sunglasses. Do not make a habit of wearing them indoors, unless you enjoy scaring waiters and small children. **TO HELP PRESERVE EYESIGHT:** Eyesight is hereditary; if your folks are four-eyes, chances are one day you will be, too. Take some sensible steps to avoid eyestrain: work and read with adequate lighting. The diffuse light from halogen lamps provides less eyestrain than glaring fluorescent lamps. If you're working at a computer screen all day, take a few 5-minute breaks. Think, listen to music, talk on the phone—and keep your eyes closed. **TO KEEP FROM CRYING:** Take a sip of water—swallowing interrupts the irregular breathing that often accompanies tears; concentrate on breathing from your belly and distract yourself with a memory of something funny or absurd.

[EYES *first aid—page 201*]

EYE MAKEUP

MANY OF THE LOOKS IN WOMEN'S MAGAZINES THAT WE ARE URGED TO EMULATE WORK UNDER A RATHER RESTRICTIVE SET OF CIRCUM- STANCES: YOU HAVE THE FLAWLESS SKIN OF AN 18-YEAR-OLD, A MAKEUP ARTIST FUSSING OVER YOU FOR TWO HOURS, A PROFESSIONAL PHOTOGRAPHER MOVING lights around until they're just so—and, oh yes, you have a photo retoucher. Most maga- zine photo layouts should be legally required to issue a warning: "Don't Try This at Home."

OPTIONS: **TO APPLY MASCARA:** Wipe wand with tissue so there's minimal goop remaining. Then, start- ing from the roots, pull the wand through the lashes, moving hand back and forth to separate lashes. After that, comb mascaraed lashes to eliminate stray clumps. **TO APPLY EYELINER:** Avoid liquid eyeliner. Apply a bit of eye powder over the eye pencil to make the line look less severe. You want the eyeliner to smudge a bit, but you don't want to look like a halfback for the Pittsburgh Steelers. **MAINTAINING EYEBROWS:** One or two models look pretty spectacular without eyebrows; the rest of us look like we just stepped off the planet Zolar. Whatever your preference, you can keep your eyebrows groomed with a stiff, slanted eyebrow brush. Apply a bit of eye shadow (in the shade of the brows) to fill in spaces you've tweezed a bit too zealously.

Regarding eyeglasses and makeup, women regularly make two mistakes when trying to adjust their makeup to their eyeglasses. If there's too little color, the eyes fade into oblivion; if the color's too aggressive, the eyes make the woman look as if she should be resting on a lily pad, scoping flies for dinner. Here are a few guidelines from makeup artist Bobbi Brown.

LIGHT-COLORED, "BLOND" GLASSES: "The overall look should be glowing and natural," says Brown. "The lips should be in soft pinks and gingers, with colors blended to the eyeglass frame. Avoid boldness. Eyelids: soft shades of red-taupe, camel, browns on lid. Liner: rich brown, coffee color, and black mascara. Eyebrows are defined, but quietly—just filled in with taupe. Blush is natural, glowing." **DARKER, "BRUNETTE" GLASSES:** "The overall look is pale, dramatic. The focus is on your lips, which should be lined and very matte, with colors in reds, cranberrys, and wines. The eye makeup should be almost nothing, just mascara and an eye shadow in a neutral caramel or café color. The brows should be strong, one shade darker than the hair—a mahogany color. Put very little color on the cheeks." **HALF-GLASSES:** "The focus is on the eyes here—if you are into eyelashes, these are the glasses for it. Make the eye smoky, outlined with pencil and dark shadow. Place charcoal or brown close to the lashes, and a bone color under the brow bone. Lips are in neutrals, a brown with red or yellow undertones, a bronze, or a caramel. The eyebrow is neither lined nor strong; the blush is tawny."

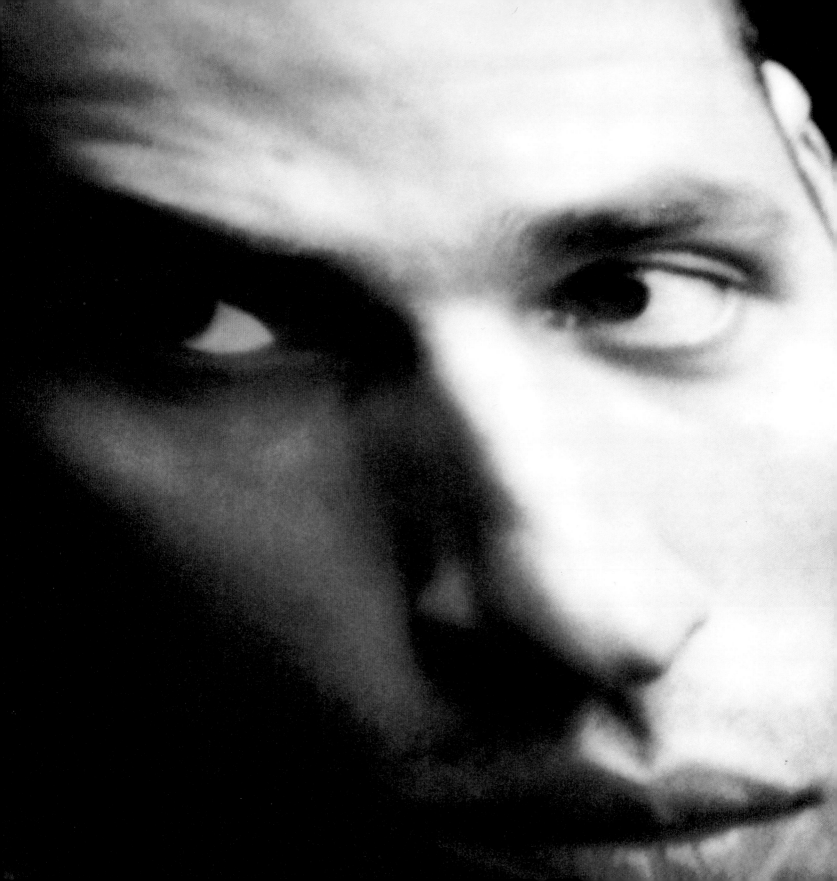

BAGS AND FOLDS

EYELID SURGERY (BLEPHAROPLASTY, AS IT'S KNOWN) IS ONE OF THE MOST COMMON, SUBTLE, AND LONG-LASTING COSMETIC PROCEDURES, ONE THAT GENERALLY LEAVES THE BEHOLDER THINKING, "HMM, SHE LOOKS GOOD. MUST BE THAT NEW HAIRCUT." AS AGE DISCRIMINATION BECOMES AN issue for men on the job as well as women, more and more men are also opting for the procedure. Removing bags under eyes erase 5 to 10 years, whether male or female.

THE PROCEDURE: Every time a muscle contracts, it wrinkles the skin. So with blepharoplasty you are in effect lifting the skin and muscle, removing superfluous pads of fat over and under the eyes (if they exist), "ironing out" the skin and redraping it, and trimming away excess. Blepharoplasty takes care of three problems: bags (fat deposits) under the eyes or over the eyelids, excessive wrinkles, and loose skin. **PAIN FACTOR:** Minimal. The operation is usually performed in the doctor's office and takes less than one hour. Stitches are removed three to four days after surgery. **HEALING:** One week to ten days after surgery, although there might be a

East meets West
Asian eyes are becoming more Westernized. There is a growing trend among Asian women to add a crease in the upper eyelid, by a process called Ssangkkop'ul, to make the eyes look wider. Interestingly, more women in Korea have this surgery performed than Korean-American women living in the United States. This kind of standardizing surgery has its detractors as well as its proponents. Vive la différence!

bit of swelling for several months. Little crosshatch marks (where the stitches were) may take several weeks to fade completely, but can be easily covered with makeup. In addition, eyes will tear for some time. Don't plan any tennis or snorkeling vacations for a month or so. **POSSIBLE COMPLICATIONS:** If too much fat is removed below the eyes, the skin wrinkles and dark shadows or circles look more prominent. If too much skin is removed from the upper eyelid, there's the chance of a slightly surprised or startled expression; too much from the bottom eyelid, where the lid is pulled downward, and the patient might end up with a "hound" droop.

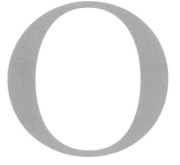

FROM CYRANO TO JIMMY DURANTE, FROM GRETA GARBO TO ANJELICA HUSTON, GREAT NOSES DEFINE A FACE. WHILE WE THINK OF EYES AS WINDOWS TO THE SOUL, THE ANCIENT GREEKS BELIEVED THE NOSE GAVE CLUES TO CHARACTER. LIKE virtually every other body part, the nose has gone through fashion cycles. The small, scooped, perky, American cheerleader nose was all the rage in the '70s; today, the ideal nose is longer, more classic, less childlike. In search of media-inspired standards of beauty, African-Americans are calling on plastic surgeons to subtly narrow their noses (while still trying to maintain their ethnicity), while Asian women are building up the bridge. But even if your nose shape doesn't conform to the ideal, it may well be the one best suited to your face.

N O

MAINTENANCE: The nose is the receptacle of smell and the entry to breathing, and keeps sunglasses on our face. It's worth taking care of.

COMBATING OIL SLICKS: The skin on the nose tends to have more oily sebaceous glands than skin on the rest of the face; hence, midafternoon shine. Be sure to rub the nose gently with a washcloth or with your hands when washing your face—this helps prevent tiny blackheads from forming by sloughing off dead skin on the nose's surface. **NOSE HAIRS:** They're extremely important for keeping bits of dust and other foreign matter out of the sinus cavities; on the other hand, they should be kept in the nose, where they belong. (Nose hairs on both men and women often grow longer with age.) Trim them with tiny clippers created especially for the purpose. **NOSE HAIR AND PLASTIC SURGERY:** Nose hairs have long been a problem primarily for men, but they've now become a problem for women after a rhinoplasty. Although a surgeon has shortened the nose and tipped it up a bit, nobody bothered to tell the nose hairs they couldn't grow as long as they used to before their home was surgically altered.

S E

[NOSE *first aid—pages 201–202*]

E A

"BIG EARS, BIG ———." AND SO GENERATIONS OF WOMEN STARED AT THE BAT EARS OF CLARK GABLE, WALTER CRONKITE, AND ROSS PEROT...AND wondered. (Of course, the same was said of feet and noses.)

"His ears make him look
like a taxicab with both
doors open."

HOWARD HUGHES *on Clark Gable*

R

S

MAINTENANCE: In youth, our ears can hear frequencies between 16,000 and 20,000 cycles per second (approximately 10 octaves) with ease; as we age and our eardrum thickens, we lose hearing at both ends of the spectrum, but particularly at higher frequencies. Thus a small loss of hearing is normal. But while we're all quick to visit the doctor if we have blurred vision, many of us ignore serious hearing loss. The reasons for the loss may be as simple as a buildup of earwax secreted in the outer ear. If you suddenly feel like you're experiencing the world while wearing an enormous pair of earmuffs, visit your doctor. **GOOD HEARING:** TURN THAT MUSIC DOWN. Got it? Stay away from Guns n' Roses concerts and construction sites—turn down the headphones. **EARWAX,** or cerumen, is the most common reason for hearing loss. It is usually simple to remove with the application of a warm oil to soften and remove the wax, but the procedure is best performed by a physician. **EAR HAIR:** As many men age, their ears tend to sprout more hair; it can be trimmed with nose-hair scissors. A popular old wives' tale says that men with hair growing out of their ears are more fertile. **EAR CREASES:** No one knows quite why, but defined ear creases in men have been linked to heart disease. If you're a guy and your ears have cleavage, better go get a checkup. **HOW TO KISS AN EAR:** Ears are highly erogenous, but only the most practiced of lovers know how to kiss them, with a caress that's feathery but not tentative. The sloppy kisser will likely make a partner shriek with laughter rather than shiver in ecstasy.

[EARS *first aid—pages 202–203*]

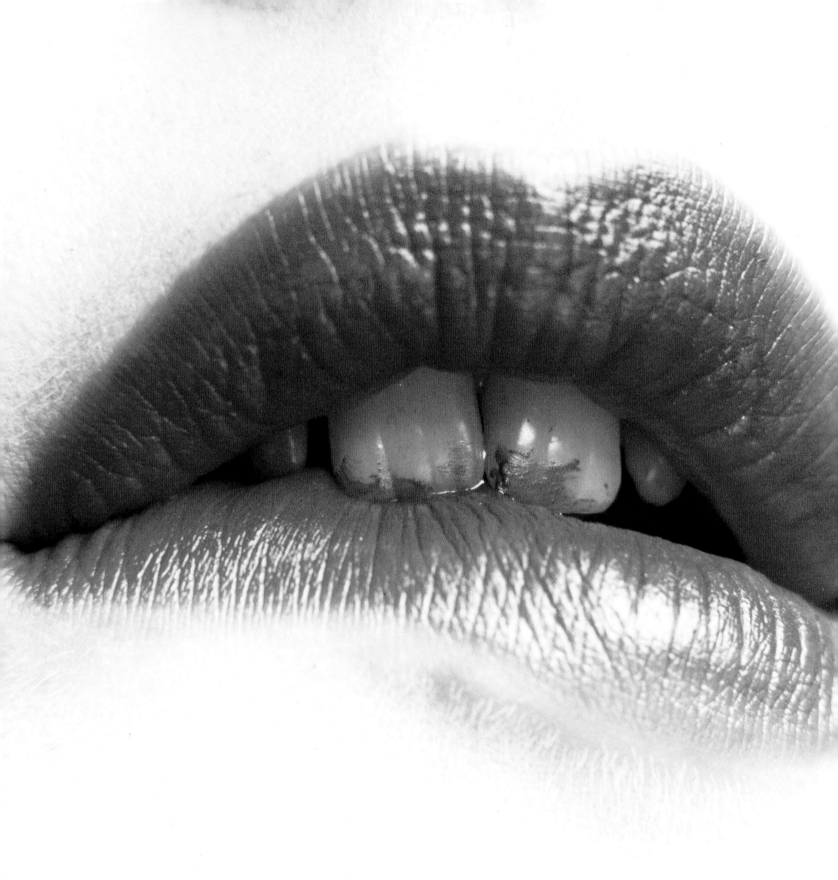

L I P S

"A KISS IS JUST A KISS," GOES THE SONG IN *CASABLANCA*—BUT IS IT? LIPS CONTAIN MEISSNER'S CORPUSCLES, SPECIALIZED EGG-SHAPED SENSORS VERY NEAR THE SKIN'S SURFACE AND OTHER AREAS (SOLES, PALMS, NIPPLES, TONGUE, PENIS, AND CLITORIS) THAT RESPOND QUICKLY TO THE LIGHTEST stimulation. Many theorists have wondered just how kissing originated. The zoologist Desmond Morris speculates that kissing began as a form of mother-to-child feeding. (Think pelicans.) Morris says, "If the young lovers exploring each other's mouths with their tongues feel the ancient comfort of parental mouth-feeding, this may help them to increase their mutual trust and thereby their pair-bonding." Or maybe it just feels right.

MAINTENANCE: **AVOIDING LIP BURN:** Lips have no melanin, which means they can't tan, but they can burn. So lips should be guarded from the sun, preferably with a lip balm that moisturizes (with petrolatum and other oils) and contains sunscreen. Use SPF protection of at least 15; the lower lip is one of the most common sites for skin cancer. **PREVENTING CHAPPED LIPS:** Brush lips regularly, and wear lip balm. Brushing lips gets rid of dead skin, and helps prevent cracking.

OPTIONS: **MATTE OR SHINY?** Blushing peach, or cherries-in-the-snow red? Full and pouting, or thin and elegant? Generally, we are drawn to lips that are red, full, and moist. Nevertheless, find what's right for you. **TO MAKE LIPS APPEAR FULLER: ALTERNATIVE 1:** Collagen or fat injections. They last up to six months, but tend to look somewhat unreal. **PREFERABLE ALTERNATIVE 2:** Invest in a lip pencil in a shade virtually the same as your own—not several shades darker. Fill in desired color.

[LIPS *first aid—pages 203*]

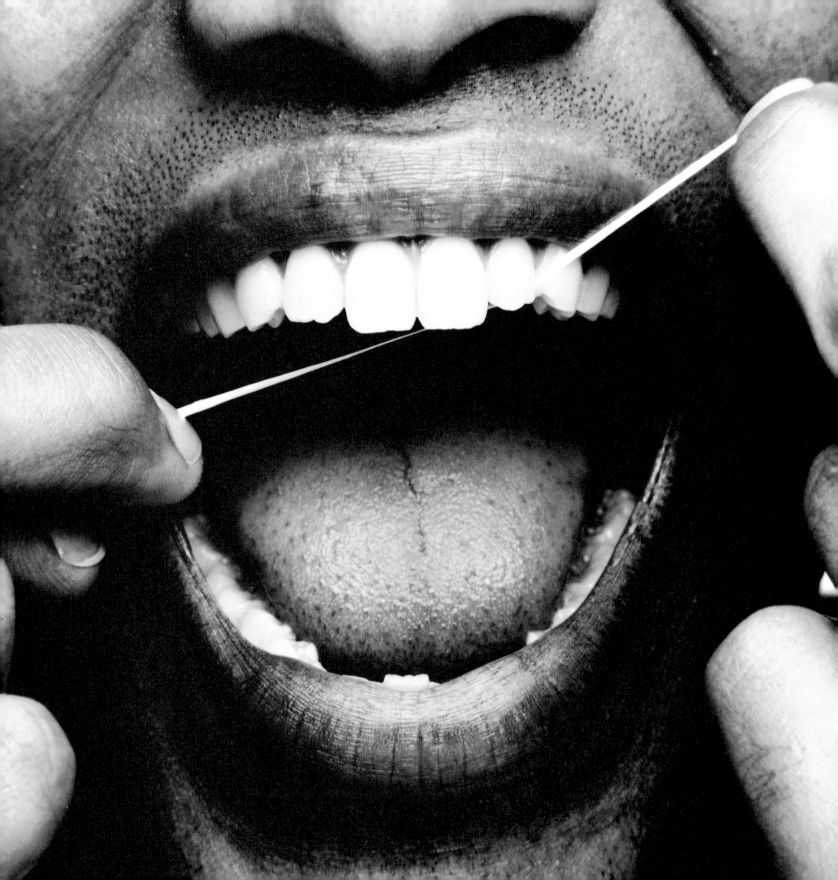

TEETH

SOMEWHERE BETWEEN GRANDMA'S SNAGGLETEETH AND THE SCARY, GLEAMING CHOPPERS OF A TV GAME SHOW HOST LIES THE PERFECT SET OF PEARLY WHITES. WE WANT TEETH WHITE, BUT NOT SO WHITE, LARGE, AND REGULAR THAT THEY LOOK FAKE; WE WANT OUR LIPS TO COVER OUR GUMS, BECAUSE a gummy smile is a goofy smile. But most of all, we want them healthy: really great teeth are about a combination of good genetics, flossing, drinking fluoridated water, and a once-every-six-months relationship with a tartar-scraping dental hygienist.

MAINTENANCE: Theories on brushing teeth keep changing. Some hygienists now say, aside from flossing, brush only the gums and go over the teeth once lightly. **AVOIDING GUM DISEASE:** Swollen, red gums that bleed when you brush or floss are early signs of gum disease, which affects more than 50 percent of the population. Gum disease is an infection caused by the plaque, or bacterial film, that coats the teeth. The key to prevention: brushing, flossing, seeing the dentist to remove hardened plaque, called tartar.

OPTIONS: **BONDING:** A kind of resin applied over enamel and between teeth to correct irregularities; think of it as Spackle for the mouth. Because teeth are not altered, bonding can be reversed—it lasts three to eight years. **PORCELAIN VENEERING:** Like bonding; but here, the dentist files down the teeth and adheres permanent laminates—veneering lasts between ten and twenty years. **BLEACHING:** There are three types of bleaching: 1) power bleaching, 2) home bleaching, and 3) over-the-counter whitening agents.

"Some tortures are physical and some are mental, but the one that is both is dental."

OGDEN NASH

[TEETH *first aid—pages 203–204*]

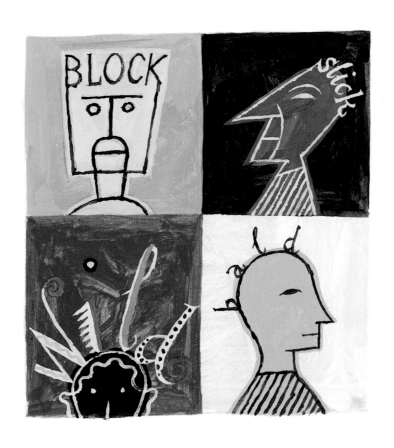

HAIR

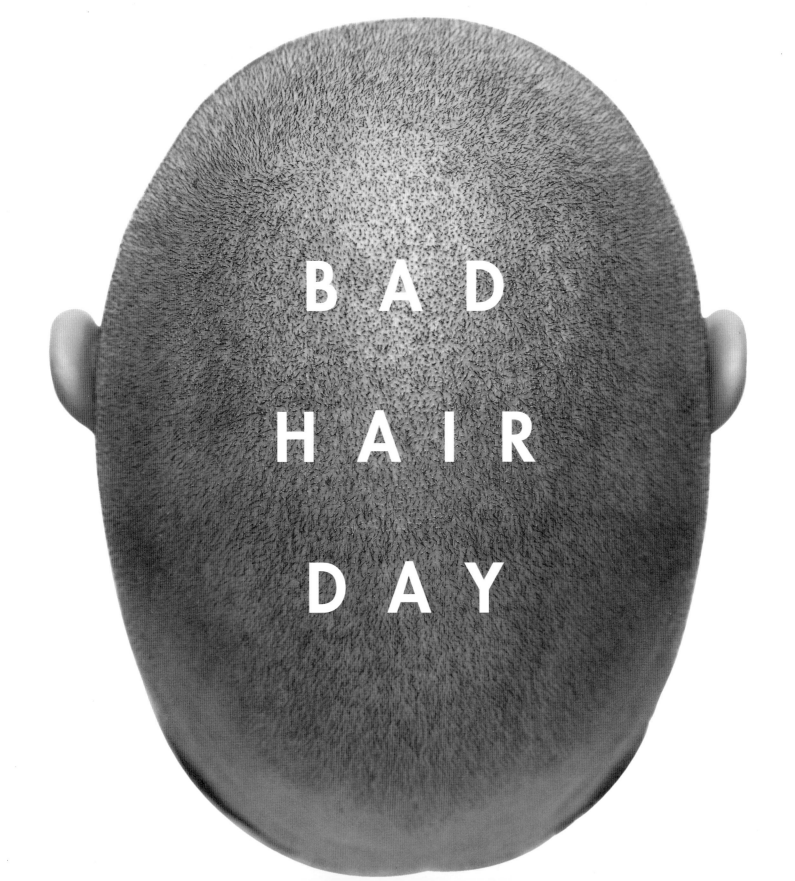

It begins with girls and their mothers, who lovingly wash and comb their hair, affixing tiny bows and ribbons when they're still almost bald. It continues throughout childhood—combing the mane on My Little Pony—and adolescence, when suddenly the state of their hair on any given day can determine whether or not they leave the house. For boys, hair fixations start somewhat later, and peak when they begin to lose it—as about one third of them do around their 35th birthday. We are a nation of the hair-obsessed. What's the point of hair? At one phase of evolutionary development, we needed our body hair to protect us against the elements. But this theory does little to explain why Inuits are not terribly hairy, while some of the hairiest people today live in some of the warmest climates. How much protection against the elements does one need in the Mediterranean? Its primary function today seems to be adornment. Odd, though, that hair can be exquisitely beautiful or hideously ugly, depending on its placement.

G R O W T H

THE AVERAGE BODY HAS ABOUT FIVE MILLION HAIRS; MERELY 100,000 OF THEM ARE ON THE HEAD. WHETHER OR NOT BLONDES HAVE MORE FUN, THEY definitely have more hair: about 140,000, as compared to 105,000 for brunettes and 90,000 for redheads. Each hair grows about two to six years; then, for a few months, its follicle goes into temporary retirement. The hair falls out, and it is eventually replaced by a new hair. Shedding 50 to 100 hairs a day is normal. From puberty until the mid-thirties hair is in its prime; estrogen plays a role not only in soft, pliable skin but in the high resistance to hair loss. One happy effect of the surge of hormones in pregnancy is the increase in the rate of hair growth, and often in its health and luster; the less happy effect is that sometimes hair growth increases all over, including lips, chin, and cheeks. Generally, excess hair falls out six months or less after giving birth. When estrogen levels begin to decline with the onset of menopause, the cells in the hair follicles begin to multiply more slowly than before—slowing down the regrowth of hair, reducing the production of sebaceous oil and pigment, and thus making the hair finer, more sparse, and often gray. A renowned hairstylist who once worked at Clairol said the company had a little rhyme: "When You Don't Know What To Do/Use No. 42." No. 42 was "Clairol Moongold," a shade referred to in the trade as "menopausal brown." So before you reach for the dye bottle, you might want to consider the possibility of not coloring— particularly if you have blue eyes and ruddy or olive skin, the ideal complexion for gray hair. Gray can be aging; it can also be beautiful.

[🖦 HAIR *first aid—pages 204–205*]

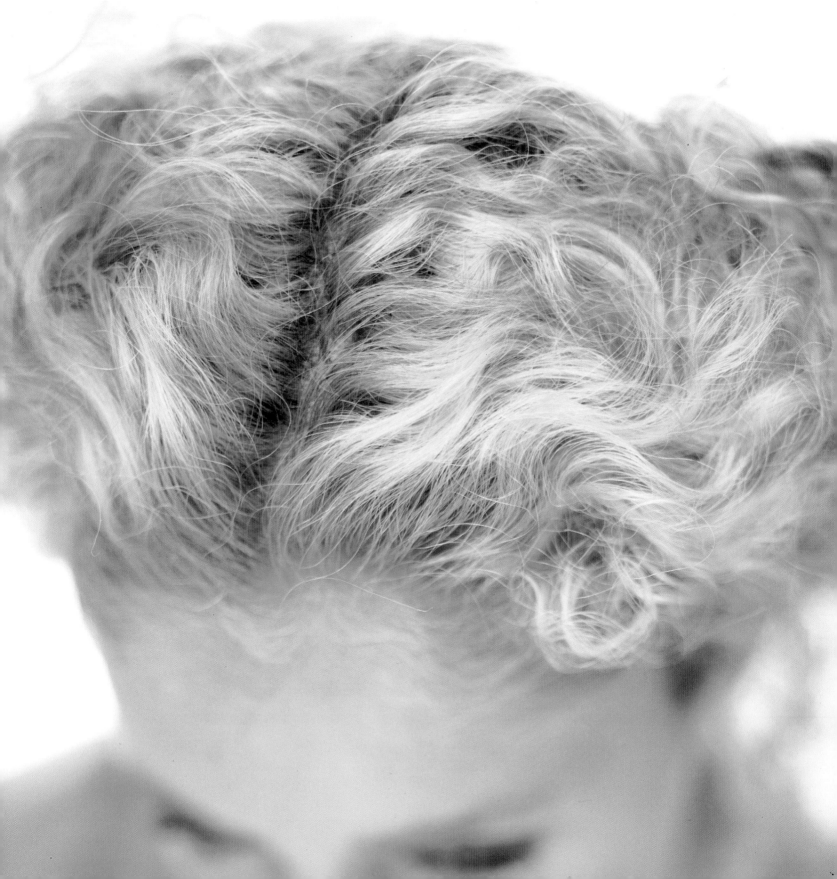

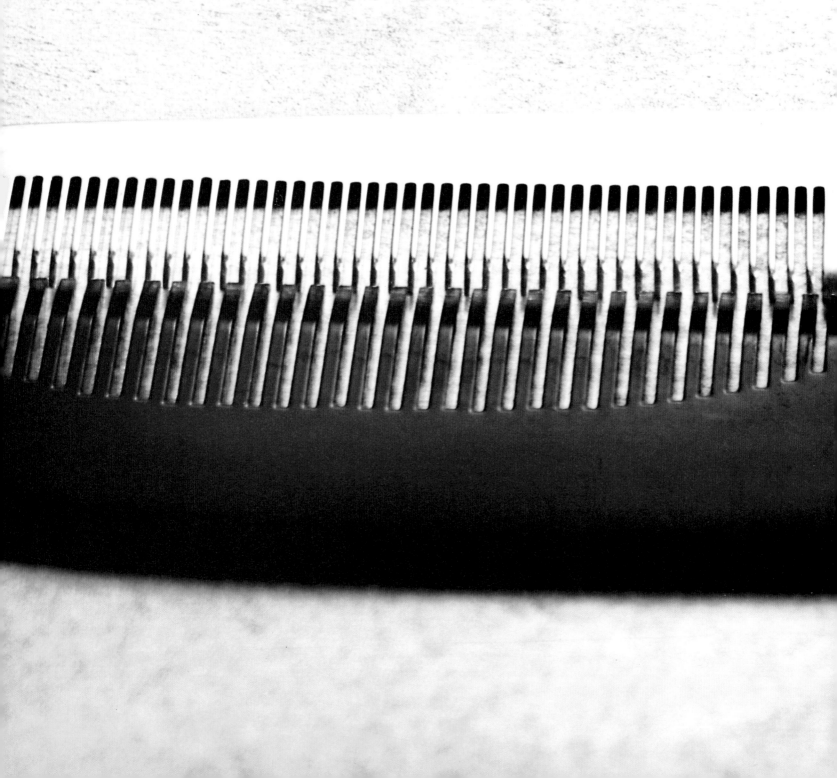

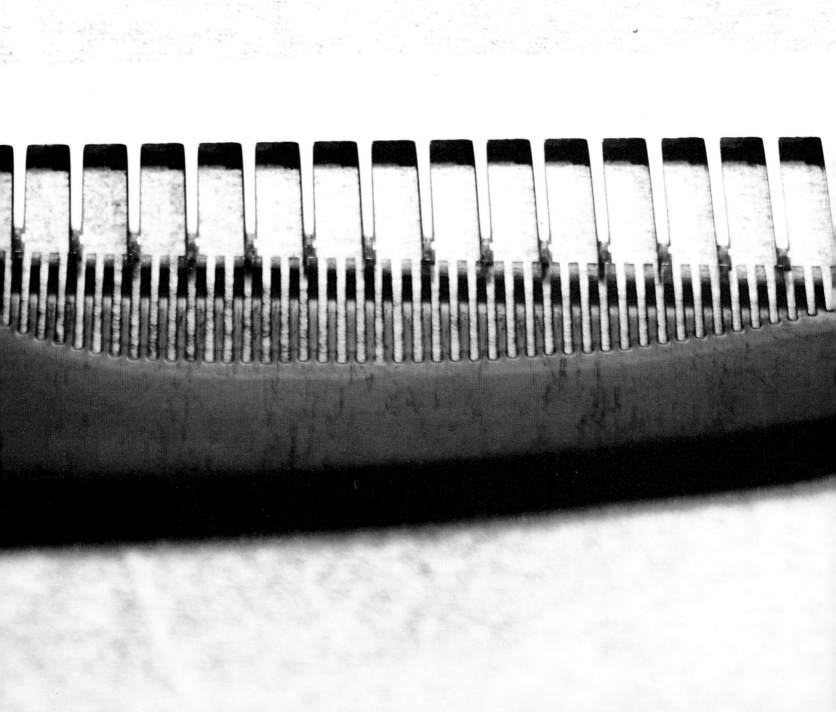

EVERYONE IS SEARCHING FOR THE UR-PRODUCT IN HAIR CARE: THE ONE SHAMPOO OR CONDITIONER THAT ABSOLUTELY WORKS. THAT PRODUCT IS—WHATEVER WORKS FOR YOU. EVEN WITHOUT A PERFECT PRODUCT, THERE ARE GUIDELINES TO KEEP HAIR HEALTHY, WHATEVER ITS TYPE OR TEXTURE: avoid excessive chlorine, saltwater, and sun exposure, particularly if hair is colored. Color-treated hair can turn a stunning shade of green in chlorinated water. The ingredients in shampoo might include everything from mint to beer, and most of them don't make a bit of difference. The only active ingredients in shampoo are its cleansers (whether they're detergents or soapless cleansers, like sodium lauryl sulfate) and its oils/humectants. Do

WASH AND

not use shampoos that make lots of lather. Lather can mean detergents. Do not shampoo hair until it's "squeaky" clean. If hair squeaks when it's clean, you may be stripping it of too much natural oil. Whatever your hair type, use a conditioner, but do not expect it to "repair" split ends. The hair cuticle, or outer layer, looks like it's made up of over-lapping scales. Conditioners and rinses temporarily fill in the space between these scales. Stearalkonium chloride is what smoothes the hair shaft: it tames the frizzies and makes hair shine. No herb or vitamin in the world will do anything without stearalkonium chloride.

MAINTENANCE: **BRUSHING OR COMBING:** Though your mother might have told you to brush your hair one hundred strokes a day, it's not such a great idea. It's too much strain on the hair, and with oily hair it may overactivate the sebaceous glands. Limit hair strokes to ten to twenty a day. **OVERCONDITIONING:** If your hair feels sticky and flat, it is possible you have overconditioned it. Solution: Detergent-based shampoo will get rid of the residue. **TO PREVENT DAN-DRUFF:** Dandruff usually results not from dry scalp (although that is possible), but from an oily scalp combined with an overgrowth of yeast microbes usually found on skin. The microbes cause irritation, inflammation, and itchiness. Medicated shampoos—containing pyrithione zinc, selenium sulfide, sulfur, salicylic acid, or tar derivatives—will generally kill the microbes. **BLOW-DRYING:** Ninety-six percent of American homes have a blow-dryer. However, remember that moisture is your hair's friend, and heat and dry air its enemy. Blow-dry as little as possible.

D R Y

Help Warning

In the Cosmetics Industry, "Help" Doesn't Help the Consumer: Whenever you see an ad that says, "X helps penetrate dry skin to moisturize," etc. this means the product doesn't actually penetrate dry skin. It helps. The word "help" is the legal loophole for getting around the fact that most cosmetics can't do exactly what advertisers claim they do. For example, no conditioner can repair damaged hair; dry, brittle hair is still dry and brittle even with a powerful humectant covering it— but the humectant makes it lie down and behave. Cosmetic ingredients only temporarily alleviate the symptoms of the problem.

"Hairstyle is the final tip-off whether or not a woman really knows herself."

HUBERT DE GIVENCHY

S T Y L I N G

IN THE NINETEENTH CENTURY, ENGLISH HAIR POMADE WAS MADE FROM BEAR GREASE; SOMETIMES LIVE BEARS WOULD BE KEPT IN BARBERSHOPS as a promotional tool to prove the pomade was fresh. Today's styling products have become somewhat tamer. Hair sprays, lacquers, shiners, gels, straighteners, mousses: whatever the formulation, the idea is to make hair easy to manage and style while still making it look like— well, like hair, and not like a furry helmet.

OPTIONS: **HAIR SPRAYS:** Early sprays contained shellac, the excretion of certain insects: it made hair shine but also made it brittle to the touch. Today, the addition of lanolin and castor oil somewhat counterbalances hair spray's ossifying effect. Tips on use: If a hairdo is not too complicated, it's better to spray it on a brush and brush it through, rather than applying directly to the head. Since fewer smog-producing ingredients, like alcohol, are being used in hair sprays, they're slower to dry. Before the final styling leave more time for hair to "set." **GELS AND MOUSSES:** Styling lotions come in two different forms. Like hair sprays, they contain copolymers that hold hair in place. But they often give greater holding power because they can be rubbed into hair, not just used to coat the outside. Depending on the strength of the copolymers, the hold can be mild or ironclad (think Day-Glo punk mohawks that wouldn't move in a wind tunnel). Tips on use: Mousses usually have a stronger hold, and are therefore better on rainy or damp days. **HAIR SHINERS:** Use liquid silicone to create shining hair (by flattening hair cuticles) and combat frizziness. **HAIR STRAIGHTENERS:** 1) Pomades coat hair and pretty much glue it straight; of all hair straighteners, these are the least effective, but also the least damaging. Great for whims. 2) Heating hair to 300 to 500 degrees and then applying tension also works; but in less than capable hands, hair snaps. 3) Various types of chemical straighteners are the most effective, but also the most potentially dangerous; scalp burns are common. Despite the popularity of at-home hair-straightening kits, straightening should be performed by a professional.

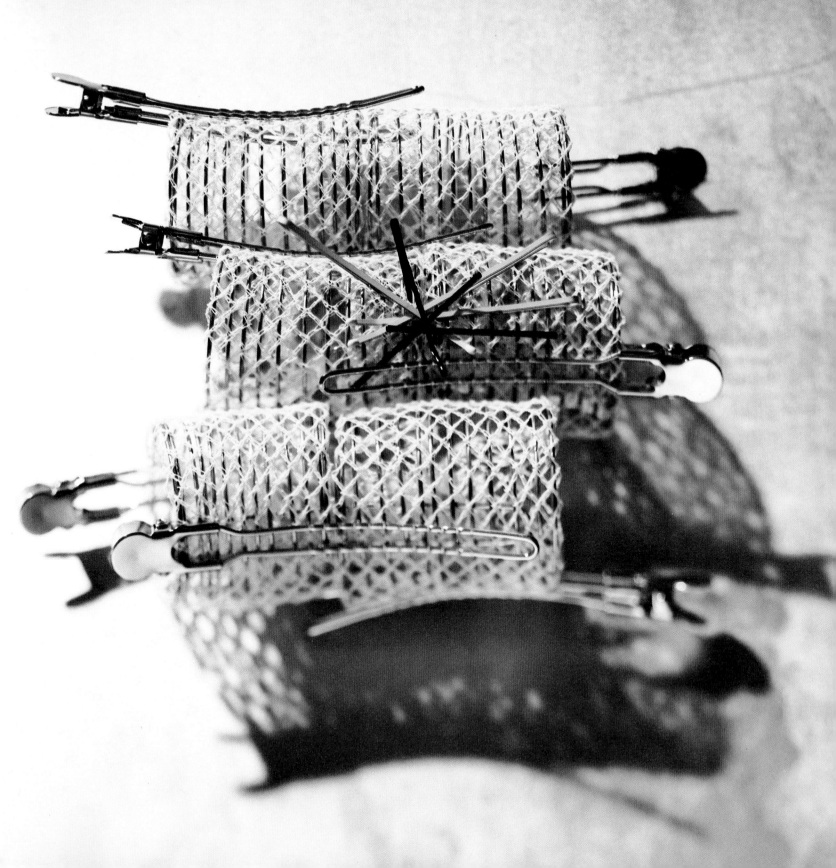

C U T

HAIR HAS ALWAYS BEEN A SOURCE OF POWER AND EROTICISM. BOTH "KAISER" AND "TSAR" MEAN "LONGHAIRED"; ORTHODOX JEWISH WOMEN SHAVE THEIR HEADS AND WEAR WIGS BECAUSE THE SIGHT OF LONG HAIR IS THOUGHT TO BE TOO SEXUALLY TEMPTING TO MEN. WHEN Delilah robbed Samson of his long locks, she stole his strength; when medieval knights rode into battle, they often wore a piece of their lady's pubic hair in a locket near their hearts. Indeed, to give some-one a lock of hair is to pledge your love, but it also gives them a certain power over you; after all, a lock of hair is often a key ingredient in witchcraft. It's no coincidence that the musical which defined the deep divide between generations during the '60s was entitled *Hair*: the way we wear our tresses has become a symbol of our beliefs and politics. When Muslims die, they're left with a single tuft of hair on their shaven heads so that Mohammed can grasp hold of them and draw them into paradise. Rastafarians regard their dreadlocks as "high-tension cables to heaven." In the '50s and '60s, a boy with a crew cut was quickly regard-ed as a pillar of society; today, that same crew cut may be regarded with deep suspicion, as it's often sported by skinheads, self-proclaimed racists, and hatemongers. Hair has become, in a sense, a metaphor for the very human desire for renewal and reinvention.

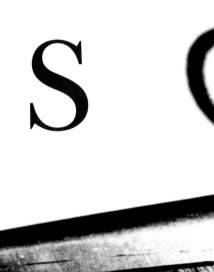

S

"A haircut is
a metaphysical
operation."

JULIO CORTÁZAR

MAINTENANCE: **FACE
TYPE:** Conventional wisdom says a
round face should be balanced with an
asymmetrical cut, a wide face with hair-
height on top for a sense of upsweep, a narrow face with fullness on the sides. That's nice
but why not ignore conventional wisdom, and
experiment with as many different styles as your
schedule, checkbook, and ego will allow. It's just hair. It
grows back. Don't sweat it. **CUTTING CYCLE:** Hairstylists
have established a Holy Law that hair should be cut every six
weeks. In fact, hair should be cut when we damn well feel like it.

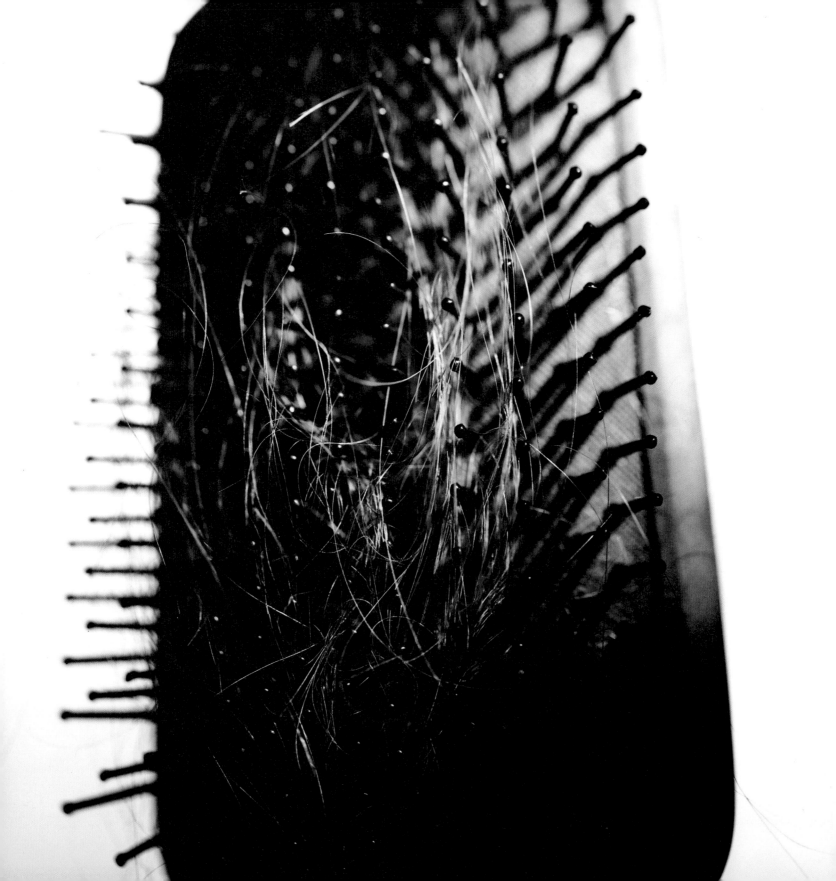

H A I R   L O S S

IN THE PANTHEON OF MALE BODILY OBSESSIONS, THE RECEDING HAIRLINE RANKS NUMBER 1 (OR, AT THE VERY LEAST, number 2, right after The Size question). Nearly two thirds of all men will eventually develop some form of balding. Still, a bald man is still a virile man—quite literally: large doses of testosterone play a role in hair loss. Hair loss for a woman can be even more devastating. While the hair loss industry has all sorts of solutions, none, at this time, are entirely satisfactory. A modest prediction: there will be a 100 percent effective solution to hair loss at about the same time they discover a 100 percent effective thigh cream.

You can comb but you can't hide

Balding men are susceptible to skin cancer on their pates, a patch of skin that's often overlooked when sunblock is applied. If a man isn't wearing a hat, he should remember to wear sunscreen: a comb-over is not protection enough.

Head today, floor tomorrow

Number of Americans afflicted by alopecia areata, a disease causing sudden hair loss ranging from quarter-sized patches to complete baldness: 2.5 million

Equal opportunity

Number of American women who experience significant hair loss: 20 million

Many Amish women suffer hair loss by constantly keeping it in a bun, thus damaging follicles.

OPTIONS: **HERE'S WHAT SCIENCE (AND ARTIFICE) CURRENTLY OFFER: MINOXIDIL** (marketed under the name Rogaine): Still the only treatment on the market that actually causes hair to grow—but, unfortunately, only for 10 to 15 percent of the people who use it, and then only for people with thinning hair. Once you start applying Minoxidil (at a cost of about $50 a month), you must stay with it forever—when treatment stops, hair falls out. **HAIR WEAVES:** Hair weaving is exactly what it sounds like—artificial hair is tied onto your remaining real hair. Weaves can be highly effective, but they can also backfire—the weave can put tension on the real hair, causing it to snap. **WIGS AND TOUPEES:** Good wigs are becoming increasingly believable and expensive (don't economize by buying fake hair). But avoid devices (wig snaps, wires, small steel spikes, velcro, crazy glue) that permanently attach to the scalp to anchor the wig—they can cause infection.

The concept of hair color has been around since the first Egyptian slapped some Nile mud on her head and noticed it turned the hair an orangey red. (Henna is, certainly, a "natural" hair dye; but just because it's natural doesn't mean it's good for you. Used alone, it leaves hair dry and brittle.) The technology of hair

coloring pretty much remained at the mud stage until the early 1900s, when several European biochemists discovered that dyes used in the manufacture of clothing, when used in conjunction with ammonia, would tint hair. Until the 1970s, the coloring process was still extremely unsophisticated: clients would have to have their hair entirely stripped of color, and then would have the tint added on top. Jean Harlow, Marilyn Monroe, and Lana Turner all

"Violet will be a good color for hai

simply had the color removed from their hair; Lucille Ball had her hair personally done by then makeup artist Max Factor, who would bleach it and add her signature tangerine shade. In the mid-'70s, products were milder and better formulated; it finally became possible to go into a top salon and become a bottle blonde, without necessarily looking like a bottle blonde. Today, color is one of the fastest-growing segments of the hair-care industry. It's not that millions of people want a radical makeover; it's the surge in graying baby boomers, on a chemically formulated search for their former— and true—selves.

OL

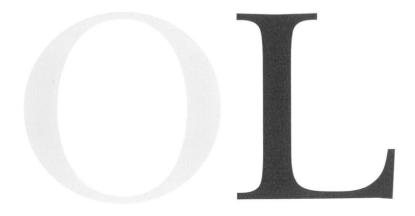

Nature's own highlights to create hair highlights without visiting the salon

For blondes, that old standby, lemon juice, mixed with equal amounts of water before putting on hair. Leave it on, sit in sun, wait.

t just about the same time that brunette becomes a good color for flowers."

FRAN LEBOWITZ

For brown or black hair, towel-dry wet hair and apply two tablespoons of molasses mixed with one tablespoon of conditioner. Work in from roots to ends. Leave on while in sun and wash out at end of day.

OR

OPTIONS: **PERMANENT TINT:** Contains ammonia, which is an enemy of hair color. **ADVANTAGE:** Hair cannot be lightened without it, because it penetrates the hair follicle and, working in tandem with bleach and peroxide, allows color to be sucked out of hair. **DISADVANTAGE:** Any product with ammonia will inevitably do some harm to hair texture. **SEMI-PERMANENT COLOR:** Contains no ammonia or peroxide, also called "developer," because manufacturers decided the word "peroxide" sounds alarming. It cannot lighten dark hair, but it can deposit color. **ADVANTAGE:** Semi-permanents do no damage. **DISADVANTAGE:** They wash out in 6 to 8 shampoos. **DEMI-PERMANENTS:** "Natural" vegetable-based dyes do contain peroxide, but no ammonia. They will not penetrate and damage the hair, nor significantly lighten it. They will deposit color, giving hair sheen. For gray heads, this process distributes the tint on both white and normal-colored hair, but it's lighter on the white hair, allowing highlights without the expensive foil process. **ADVANTAGE:** A demi-permanent lasts about 30 to 40 shampoos, and gives hair a natural gloss. Demi-permanents are so gentle that you can get your hair colored and permed on the same day. **DISADVANTAGE:** Demi-permanents are ineffective if you're determined to go lighter.

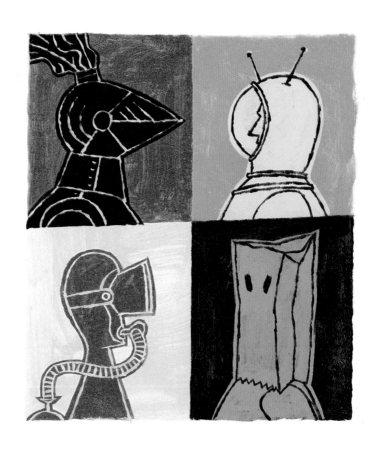

SKIN

"Oh, the white folks hate the black folks, And the black folks hate the white folks... And the Hindus hate the Moslems, and everybody hates the Jews."

TOM LEHRER

The only thing that's dated about Tom Lehrer's 1960s ditty "National Brotherhood Week" is that he left out a few groups: blacks vs. Koreans in New York, Cubans vs. blacks in Miami, whites vs. Chicanos in Los Angeles—and skinheads vs. everybody who's not a skinhead. Today, as South Africa is slowly, painfully breaking the chains of apartheid, our country seems to be facing some of the most racially heated times since Selma. Tune into a daytime talk show, and likely

DOES MY SKIN FIT

as not a black woman and a white woman will be facing off. To say that skin color or religion is the only thing separating us is reductive and naive. We are separated by class and money and beliefs and—perhaps most sadly—aspirations. This chapter of the book is simply about skin—its physical properties, its care and feeding. But it doesn't hurt to remember that in the wider world, when it comes to color, something has gone wrong here that's more than skin deep.

E X P O S U R E

SKIN IS OUR LARGEST ORGAN, AND ANYONE WHO DOUBTS JUST HOW SENSITIVE THIS ORGAN IS NEED ONLY SPEND one day getting a sunburn on a nude beach. Most Americans understand that sun exposure prematurely ages skin. They also know exposure to the sun's ultraviolet rays increases the chance of skin cancer by damaging immune response, weakening the skin's ability to fight abnormal cells. Changing our knowledge and changing our psyches are two different things. Sixty-six percent of Americans still think tans "look healthy," and 33 percent work hard to get a tan. If you can't resist, use a sunscreen which can handle not only UVB rays, which cause burning, but also some UVA rays, which accelerate skin wrinkling and aging.

O P T I O N S : **SUNSCREENS VS. SUNBLOCKS:** Sunscreens chemically absorb the sun's rays, but unfortunately some people are irritated by sunscreen chemicals. Those people should use sunblocks, which have an SPF of 15 or higher and use microscopically ground-up metals like titanium dioxide to reflect the sun's rays like a mirror. **THE HIGHER THE SPF, THE BETTER?** While SPFs (sun protection factors) of 2 or 4 may be ineffective on fair skin, SPFs of above 30 are unnecessary, and may cause skin irritation. **RETIN-A AND THE SUN:** Although Retin-A repairs sun-damaged skin, the cream's skin-thinning properties also make those same rejuvenated complexions much more susceptible to sun damage—you MUST stay out of the sun.

Why you don't want to even think about not using sunscreen

Number of new cases of skin cancer (all types) in the U.S. in 1991: 632,000

Increase since 1985: 50%

Percentage of adults who use sunscreen: 41%

Percentage who stay out of the sun altogether: 26%

Percentage decrease in skin-cancer risk among those who avoid the sun vs. those who don't: 97%

Why sunblock is really, really important

Number of Americans who have gone skinny-dipping: 23 million (about 1 in 10)

Number of nude beaches in America: 200

[🗒 SKIN *first aid—pages 205–206*]

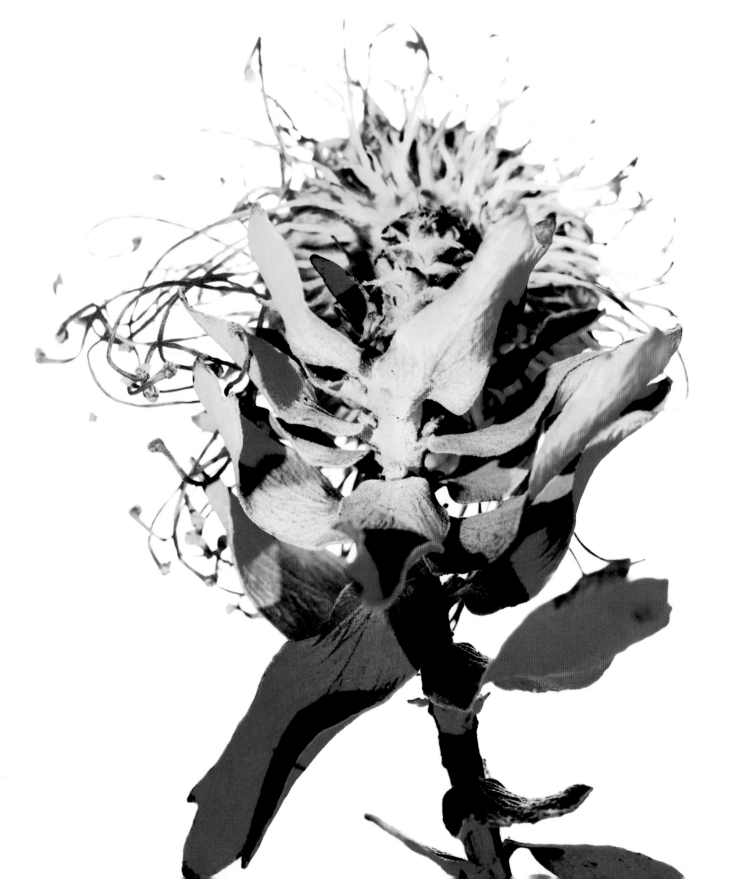

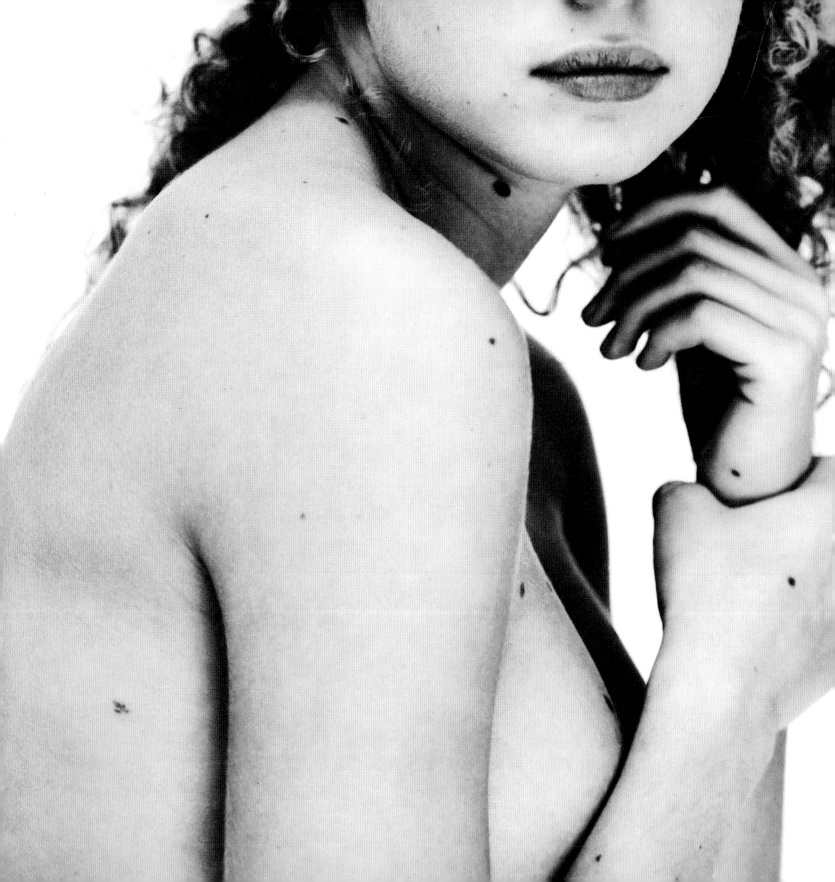

S P O T S

REMEMBER YOUR COUSIN EDNA AT THE FAMILY REUNION? REMEMBER THAT MOLE ON HER NOSE THAT GAVE YOU NIGHTMARES FOR years? How did freckles—those brownish or yellowish concentrations of melanin on the skin—become cute, while moles (which may look like freckles, but are usually raised on the skin) become scary? (Unless, of course, they're moles above the lips of Marilyn Monroe or Cindy Crawford—then they're called beauty marks, and they're sexy.) Well, there may be some medical reasons for our folkloric prejudices: though most moles are harmless, these growths must be monitored. New moles—or any that change in size, shape, or color or that bleed—could indicate skin cancer and should be examined by a doctor.

MAINTENANCE: For those who want to be a bit less spotty. **LIVER SPOTS:** These flat, brown marks appear as we age; they're actually areas of increased pigmentation, brought on by years of exposure to the sun. They can be removed either with a prescription bleaching preparation, a laser, or a light chemical peel. Liver spots can also be lightened with Retin-A. **MOLES:** Suspicious moles can easily be removed, either by shaving them off the skin surface with a scalpel or, for those with roots, by cutting them out. **SKIN TAGS:** These tiny chunks of excess skin are generally harmless; they develop as a result of heredity, aging, pregnancy, or friction in skin folds. The best treatment is scissor removal: the dermatologist numbs the skin and snips them off. **SEBORRHEIC KERATOSES:** These dark, wartlike growths generally appear on parts of the body rarely exposed to the sun. A doctor can remove them with liquid nitrogen. **SOLAR KERATOSES:** Normally the result of sun exposure, these are usually precancerous; they start off as a pink or slightly raised patch, then progress to a scaly red or brown lesion. They can be scraped off by a physician or treated with Retin-A. **FACIAL WARTS:** These are viral growths often looking like seborrheic keratoses. They spread easily, and should be removed quickly.

S C R U B

THE KEY TO SMOOTH SKIN IS WASHING WITH SOAP TO REMOVE DIRT AND BACTERIA, EXFOLIATING—REMOVING THE OUTER LAYER OF DEAD SKIN CELLS—WITH A LOOFAH OR WASHCLOTH (USE GENTLE CIRCULAR MOTIONS), AND COVERING THE BODY WITH MOISTURIZER. That's it. Fragrance of soap, price, color, exotic plant or mineral extract, etc., is up to you.

MAINTENANCE: No matter how much you enjoy a good wallow, limit your time in the bath to twenty minutes a day. Any more will dry your skin. **EFFECTIVENESS:** There's really no correlation between the price of a moisturizer and its ability to moisturize. Cheaper products use slightly cheaper ingredients that may not feel as pleasant as their high-end counterparts. Many use that old standby, glycerin, to trap moisture in the skin instead of hyaluronic acid, which would give a lighter, more evanescent texture to the cream. **COST:** Additionally, as much as 60 percent of the cost of any cosmetic product is in the packaging—so the packaging of less expensive products may not look as pretty perched on your shelf, but they can be just as effective on your skin.

"The body says what words can-not."

MARTHA GRAHAM

OPTIONS: Thanks to our interest in maintaining our skin, the spa industry is growing faster than you can say "thalassotherapy." **MUD BATHS:** Mud is nothing more than clay or sand and water with traces of minerals—sulfur, calcium, magnesium, fluoride. Slathered on the skin, it acts as an astringent, drawing out oil, bacteria, and dirt. **SEAWEED WRAPS:** The latest in mineral treatments is thalassotherapy, where the bather is dipped in seawater and wrapped in mineral-rich seaweed. You don't need to buy commercial products. Simply soak dried seaweed, such as kombu, and apply the slippery gel to your skin. The seaweed temporarily smoothes skin; some claim that vitamins and minerals, applied topically, have antioxidant properties.

[SCRUB *first aid—page 206*]

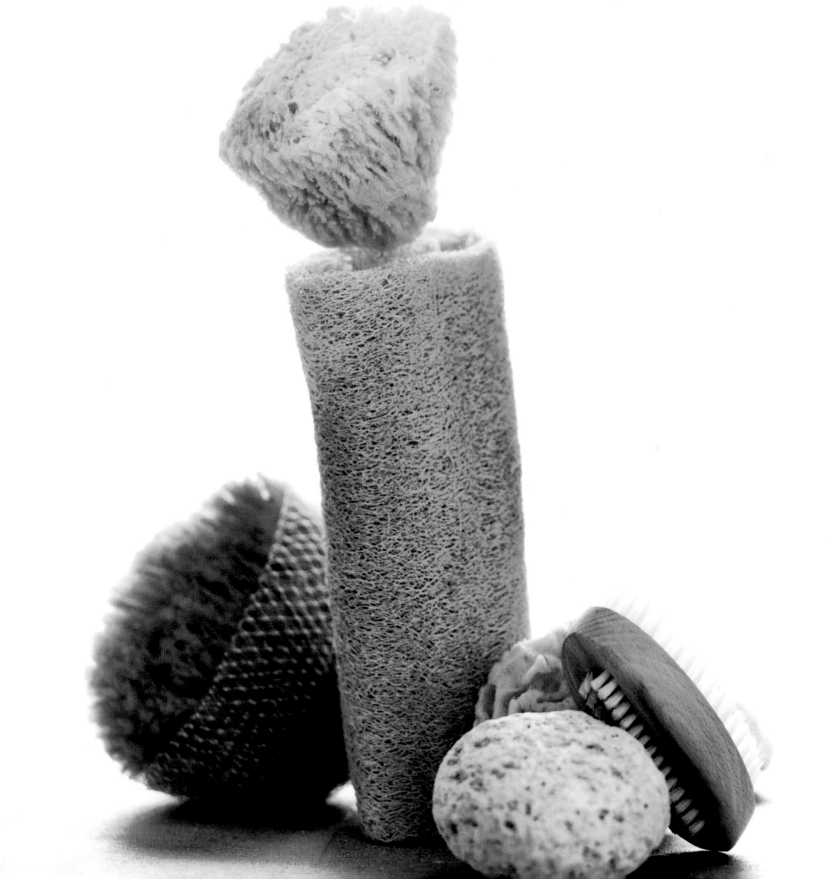

AMERICA IS OBSESSED WITH FEMALE BODY

HAIR; WOMEN HAVE JUST AS MUCH HAIR ON THEIR

BODIES AS MEN, YET WE WANT THEM AS SMOOTH AND HAIRLESS

AS PREPUBESCENTS. SOME FEMINISTS THINK THIS IS EMBLEMATIC

of our society's depraved need to keep women in a childlike state. Unfortunately,

many of us who otherwise strive to uphold feminist values are wussies when it comes to

body hair. We shudder at the crushed-spider-under-glass look of hairy legs under nude

stockings. No sophisticated Frenchwoman with armpits like a wolverine is going to

convince us it's not ugly. For the non-Continental, here are some hair-removal guidelines:

OPTIONS: **SHAVING:** ADVANTAGES: Quick, cheap, easy, painless. DISADVANTAGES: Very short-term; hair starts growing back immediately. The Mediterraneans among us suffer from five o'clock leg shadow. HOW TO: Use a shaving cream or gel; sit in water long enough to soften and swell hairs. **DEPILATORIES:** ADVANTAGES: Painless, cheap, lasts slightly longer than shaving. Works by chemically dissolving hair slightly below skin surface. DISADVANTAGES: Messy, time-consuming, can be irritating to the skin, smells like nothing else on earth. HOW TO: Follow directions on bottle, making sure to test a patch of skin first to make sure the depilatory doesn't make it red or itchy. Wash off in shower. **HAIR BLEACHING:** ADVANTAGES: Also painless and cheap; does not remove hair, but makes it less noticeable against light skin. DISADVANTAGES: Messy, time-consuming; if skin is dark, bleached hair looks too yellow, thus enhancing the hair problem instead of minimizing it. HOW TO: Follow directions for mixing bleach and "activator" granules. WARNING: It doesn't require a degree in chemistry to mix the bleach formula, but this stuff irritates skin if left on too long or not mixed properly. **WAXING:** ADVANTAGE: Rips hair from the root, resulting in much longer regrowth rate; leaves skin silken and smooth. Repeated waxings seem to make hair grow back more sparsely. DISADVANTAGE: Hurts. A lot. HOW TO: Forget about home leg-waxing kits, unless you've been using them since the days you played with Barbie. Go to a salon. To reduce the chance of ingrown hairs after waxing (curlyheads are particularly susceptible), massage waxed area with a loofah to keep pores open. WARNING: Do not use wax on any skin areas on which you've used Retin-A. **ELECTROLYSIS:** ADVANTAGE: The only truly permanent method of hair removal. A disposable needle probes the hair follicle and kills it with a tiny electric current. DISADVANTAGE: Pain-wise, it makes waxing seem like a soothing massage. Additionally, it's expensive and time-consuming; sometimes a hair follicle needs to be zapped often.

S C E

"NOTHING AWAKENS A REMINISCENCE LIKE AN ODOR," VICTOR HUGO ONCE WROTE, AND HE MIGHT HAVE ADDED THAT THE OPPOSITE HOLDS TRUE: AN ODOR CAN BE AWAKENED BY A REMINISCENCE. THINK BACK TO KINDERGARTEN, and you're likely to smell that rich, earthy scent of Play-Doh. The years tick by with the smells: junior high is mimeograph paper; high school is the acrid whiff of marijuana; college is a first lover whose sweat-drenched body spoke to you in the language of pheromones, those mysterious scents of attraction. Whereas sight objectifies, smell subjectifies: our visceral reactions to smells force us to become

N T

participants, while vision keeps us at a distance from the object of our attention, making us observers. Smell can be terrifying, because it works at the most primitive level, divorced from logic or calculation. Lillian Hellman recalled how her first love said he didn't like the way she smelled. She claimed she never recovered from this slight. Smell, more than any other sense, is imbued with deep ambivalence. America is terrified of natural odors. To hear Madison Avenue tell the story, Americans feel about human odor as they do about tax audits: a necessary evil, but one that should happen to someone else.

Fragrance
Since earliest times, people haven't wanted to smell like themselves, despite the evidence of the appeal of pheromones. Fragrances are composed using the principle of three notes: top, base, and middle. More than one ingredient from each group may be used to make a single scent. Some perfumes include hundreds.

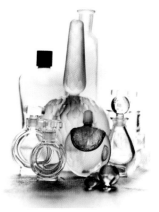

Fragrance glossary
The difference among various types of fragrance is *strength*: the lower the ratio of perfume to alcohol, the more long-lasting the fragrance.
Perfume:
5 to 6 hours
Cologne:
2 to 3 hours
Toilet water:
2 to 3 hours
Perfume in lotion:
3 to 4 hours
Aftershave:
2 to 3 hours

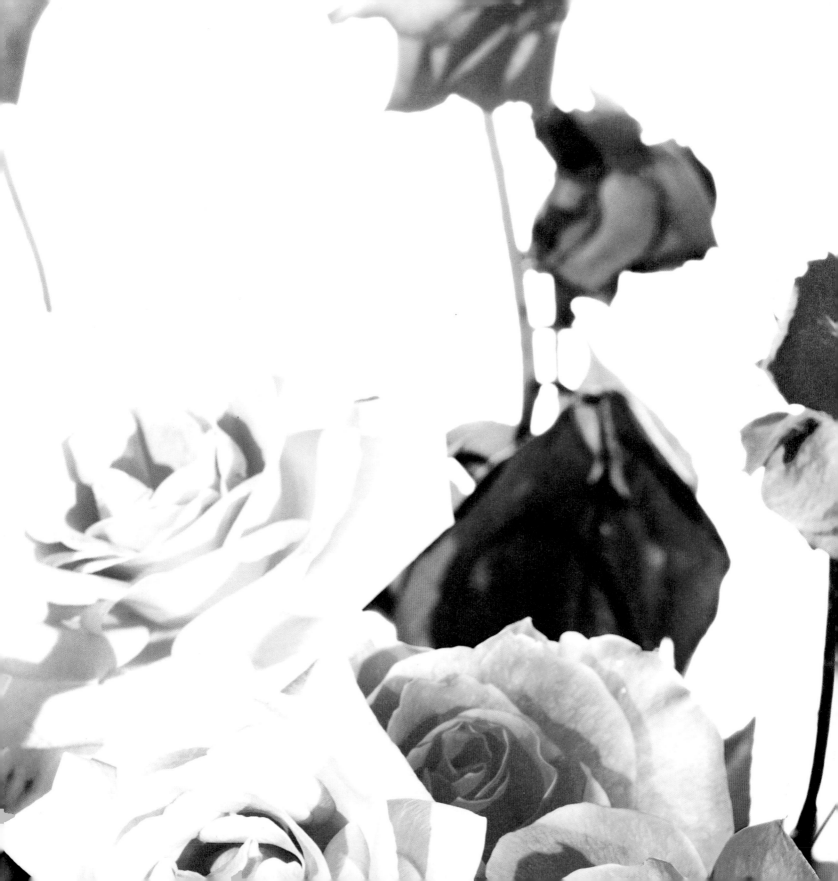

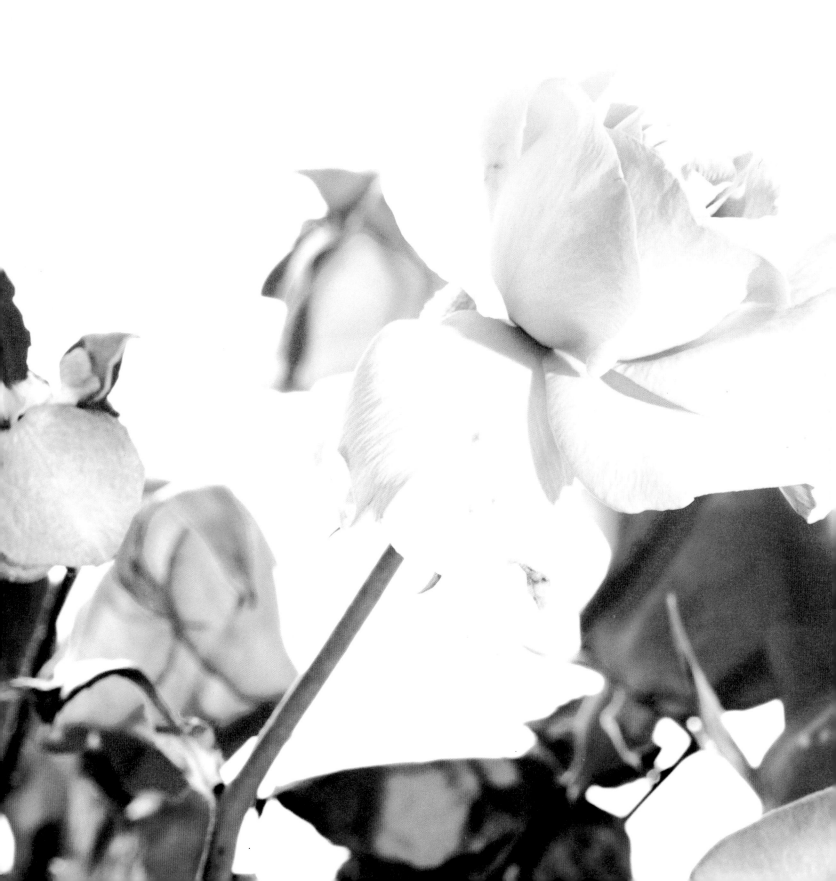

ADORNMENT

TATTOOS: Once tattoos were the province of bikers and prisoners with too much time on their hands; next they were on the ankles and shoulders of the fashion world. Tattoos can even be used to disguise and enhance scars. An L.A. writer had her mastectomy scar transformed into a multicolored vine trailing delicately across her chest. According to tattoo artists, today about four out of ten clients are now women—and not your average motorcycle mamas either.

BODY PIERCING: Remember when getting your ears pierced was a challenge to your parents' authority? Body piercing is nothing new: dozens of cultures have regarded piercing and scarification as rites of passage. Piercing and tattooing are additional decisions about adorning your body, but unlike with a new haircut, the end result is not as transient. Remember, models and celebrities often don fake tattoos and faux pierced jewelry that only last as long as the photo shoot.

MAINTENANCE: **REMOVING TATTOOS (AT LEAST PARTIALLY):** These days tattoos can be removed by lasers: the pulse of light breaks up black, blue, and green pigments embedded in the skin. The ink particles are carried off into the bloodstream, with no anesthetic needed. But there are still no completely satisfactory methods of tattoo removal. **BODY PIERCING:** Pierced ears heal within a few days; other body parts do not. Lips take about six weeks to heal, nostrils six to nine months. And you don't even want to know about nipples. But if you're hell-bent on piercing, make sure the needle is sterilized, because infections develop rather easily. If you do get an infection, ask your doctor for some surgical scrub disinfectant to use on the sore—alcohol is too harsh, and antibiotic ointments keep air from getting in and healing the wound. Finally, always wear stainless steel, silver, or gold jewelry—never cheap off-the-street stuff, because junk jewelry makes the pierced site even more likely to become infected.

"I attribute my whole success in life to a rigid observance of the fundamental rule—never have yourself tattooed with any woman's name, not even her initials."

P. G. WODEHOUSE

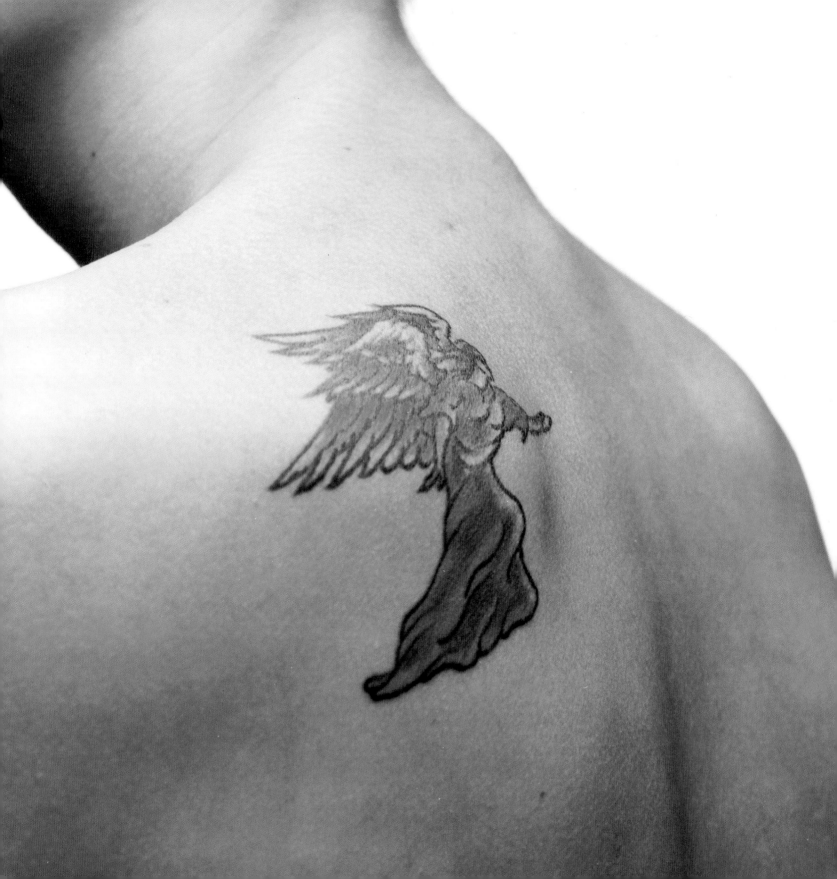

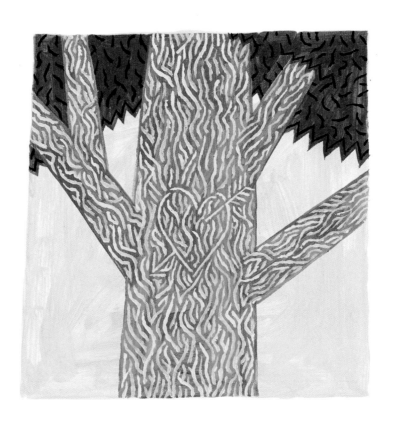

TORSO

IS MY CENTER

CENTERED

The solar plexus, a complex of nerves at the pit of the stomach, is so named because it's the area from which our energy, our life-force, radiates. An essential quality for any athlete is a low center of gravity; for example, no matter how bulging the biceps of a weight lifter, he won't be capable of lifting much more than wussy weights if his abs and glutes aren't equally well developed. A surfer must find her center with eyes closed and heart pounding; an astronaut learns the secret of staying balanced without gravity—when up is not up and down is not down. When Eastern science talks about the chakras, they're talking about the seven areas of the body from which energy flows; one of the vital chakras is located right smack in the middle of the gut—in fact, in the solar plexus. Do you feel you need to be connected to the earth, "centered"? A crystal healer would advise you to meditate with a chunk of green malachite over your loins. Of course, the rest of us might just go hiking, or do a lot of sit-ups.

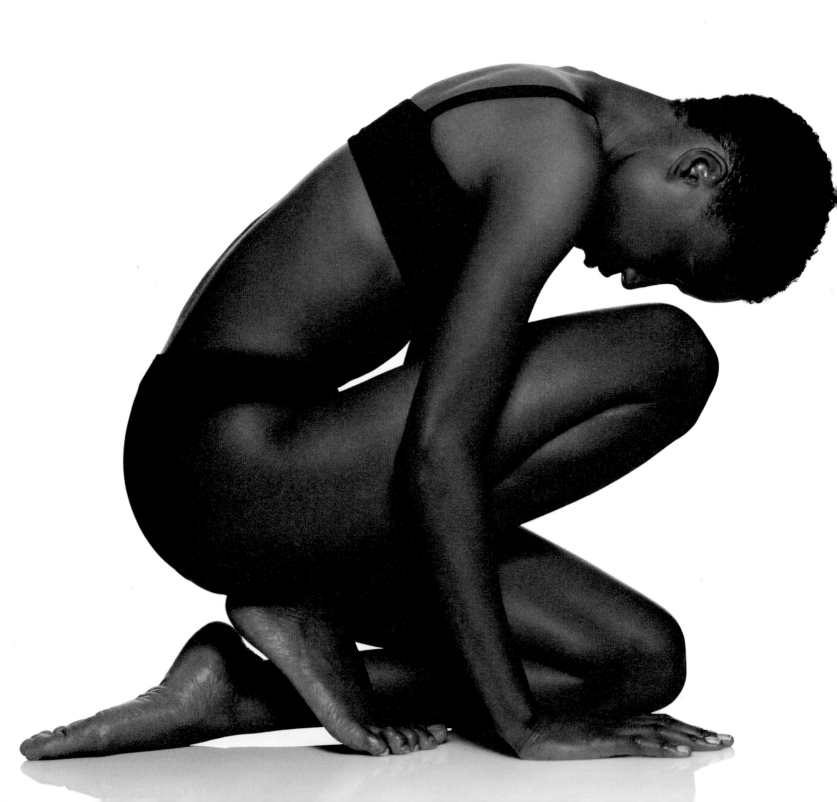

SHOULDERS

WHAT'S AT THE BOTTOM OF THE FEMALE (AND SOMETIMES MALE) CONFESSION "I CAN'T RESIST A MAN IN UNIFORM"? WHAT WE ASSOCIATE WITH that uniform is certainly not the cut of the cloth, or the fact of a man in other-than-civilian dress. (You don't hear too many women cooing, "I can't resist a man in a clown suit.") It's that quality of carriage a uniform brings, summed up in the phrase "military posture." In our culture, rounded shoulders reflect weakness and vulnerability, while square shoulders bespeak confidence and power. Politicians work hard, sartorially, to convey this tacit message; no matter how round their shoulders may actually be, the same shoulders in a suit look perfectly square. Amazing what a little padding will do.

MAINTENANCE: Ever notice that a toddler doesn't slouch? Bad posture is mostly a result of stomach and back muscles that have weakened with time. Maintaining good posture as we get older may help alleviate back problems, and also creates a satisfying optical illusion: merely standing tall makes one look ten pounds lighter and, strangely, creates an outward sense of self-confidence. **AVOID SCHLEPPING:** Over the long haul, carrying a laptop or heavy pocketbook slung over one shoulder will throw shoulders out of alignment and encourage slovenly posture. If possible, distribute carried weight evenly, perhaps in a backpack. **EXERCISE TO STRENGTHEN ROUNDED SHOULDERS:** Stand holding weights, with arms raised to shoulder height and palms facing front. Slowly bring weights together directly over head, and then back down to shoulder height, 10 to 15 times. Repeat set 3 times. Perform this exercise every other day, and in about two months you'll begin to see changes. **DECORATE:** When showing our shoulders, there's a fine line between alabaster skin on the neck and shoulders and halibut-belly white; those of us who lean toward halibut can cover blue veins peeping through with a cream foundation or powder, or perhaps a sunless tanning lotion.

CHEST

REMEMBER THOSE COMIC-BOOK DRAWINGS

OF THE 90-POUND WEAKLING WHO WAS FOREVER

GETTING SAND KICKED IN HIS FACE? THE PART OF HIS BODY

SINGLED OUT FOR SCORN WAS INVARIABLY HIS PIGEON CHEST—

PARTICULARLY AS COMPARED TO THE BULLY'S HUGE EXPANSE OF RIPPLING

muscle. This is the image little boys in our culture have had to live with. And this yearn-

ing is not unsupported by the gaze of female admirers: a man's chest is, according to some

studies, the third physical characteristic a woman notices about a man, right after eyes and

buttocks. Hairy or hairless is a matter of taste, but it seems women prefer one or the other—

there's a certain aversion to a few meek sprouts of hair trying pathetically to burst forth.

OPTIONS: PUMPING UP: "We must, we must, we must increase our bust." Such was the mantra of flat-chested 12-year-old girls. But men really can expand the width of their chests through any exercise that works the upper body—swimming, weight lifting, gardening. The idea is to keep the chest muscles from atrophying and sagging as we age. **CHEST AND SHOULDER HAIR REMOVAL:** More and more men are opting to remove body hair, through shaving or (for the truly deranged) waxing. The reason most often cited? Muscle definition: men who take all that time working out don't want those pumped pecs to be lost in a forest of hair. **CHEST WIGS:** They exist. Some men wear them. Enough said. **GYNECOMASTY:** Sometimes hormonal changes with age or sudden weight gain can leave men with extra fatty tissue in the breast. With a gynecomasty, the most common cosmetic surgical procedure among men, excess fat tissue is removed to create a harder, flat look. **PECTORAL IMPLANTS:** Some men are turning to pectoral implants to create that brawny look without all the work. Actually, a scrupulous plastic surgeon will insist a candidate for this surgery try an exercise regimen first. Under general anesthesia, an incision is made under the axilla and up to three five-inch solid silicone implants are placed under the chest muscle, the pectoralis major. The chest is then tightly wrapped for about a week and the patient can become active again in three weeks when scar tissue holds everything in place. **PROBLEMS:** Possible complications include infection, bleeding, or slippage of the implants—in which case they would be repositioned. Makes exercise look good.

"[Dieting and cosmetic to work very well, at least work at the same time. thing intrinsically wrong dangerous or helpful, content and our motive— reach the image in

G L O R I A

Just when we thought we had heard enough about the "S" word.... Feminist Gloria Steinem's recent *Revolution from Within* tackles the problem of low self-esteem—her own and women's in general. One particularly pervasive symptom in our society: poor body image. "I never questioned the wrongness of my body image until I was in my thirties and saw myself on television. There was this thin, pretty, blondish woman of medium height.... This was a shock. What I felt like *inside* was a plump

surgery] don't seem
not without serious inner
It isn't that there is any-
with them—each may be
depending on its
but ultimately, they don't
our mind's eye."

STEINEM

brunette from Toledo, too tall and much too pudding-faced." Steinem is apparently far from alone in this: she cites many studies in which women of all ages consistently rated themselves fatter and uglier than they, in fact, were. (Men, on the other hand, consistently rate themselves both thinner and better-looking than they actually are.) So, while Steinem takes an uncharacteristically laissez-faire attitude on dieting and cosmetic surgery in general, she warns against substituting them for work on poor self-esteem.

WHEN DOES THE OBSESSION START? IS IT THE DAY
GIRLS START PLAYING WITH BARBIE AND WONDER WHY THEIR
CHESTS DON'T LOOK LIKE THAT? IN STUDY AFTER STUDY, WOMEN WITH
LARGE BREASTS ARE DISPROPORTIONATELY PERCEIVED AS MORE SEXY—AND
stupider—than women with smaller breasts. Breasts have been eroticized to the point where
we've lost a sense of their original purpose. How else to explain that magazines can sport
ads picturing bare-breasted women, yet public breast-feeding is illegal in some states?

BREAST

"Don't eat too many almonds; they add
weight to the breasts."

COLETTE, *Gigi*

MAINTENANCE: Nationwide, one out of ten women will be diagnosed as having breast cancer. Risk factors include: more than one family member who has had breast cancer; a high-fat diet; smoking combined with using the Pill; not having a first pregnancy before the age of 35. Scientists are still not sure why breast cancer is more common today than it was in our mothers' generation. Which is why a yearly mammogram after the age of 35, and a monthly breast self-examination, is more than merely advisable—it's necessary. **MINIMIZING SWELLING:** Some women swear by a daily folic acid supplement before their period; most of us just need to cut down on our favorite fluid-retainers, caffeine and salt.

OPTIONS: For those who think size counts: **BREAST AUGMENTATION:** A relatively simple surgical procedure, in which a pouch of saline solution or silicone is inserted in front of the muscle tissue of the breast. Recently, the FDA banned silicone breast implants for cosmetic use because of the dangers of autoimmune reaction—there's been no proof that the incidence of autoimmune reaction is any greater in the breast-implant population than in the regular population. **REDUCTION:** Women, generally, are less enthusiastic than men about mammoth breasts: all that weight can cause poor posture and chronic back pain. In breast-reduction surgery, fatty tissue is excised and the nipple moved to position it properly on the new, smaller models; the result may be less nipple sensitivity. Some women also lose the ability to breast-feed. As in all things, think about it.

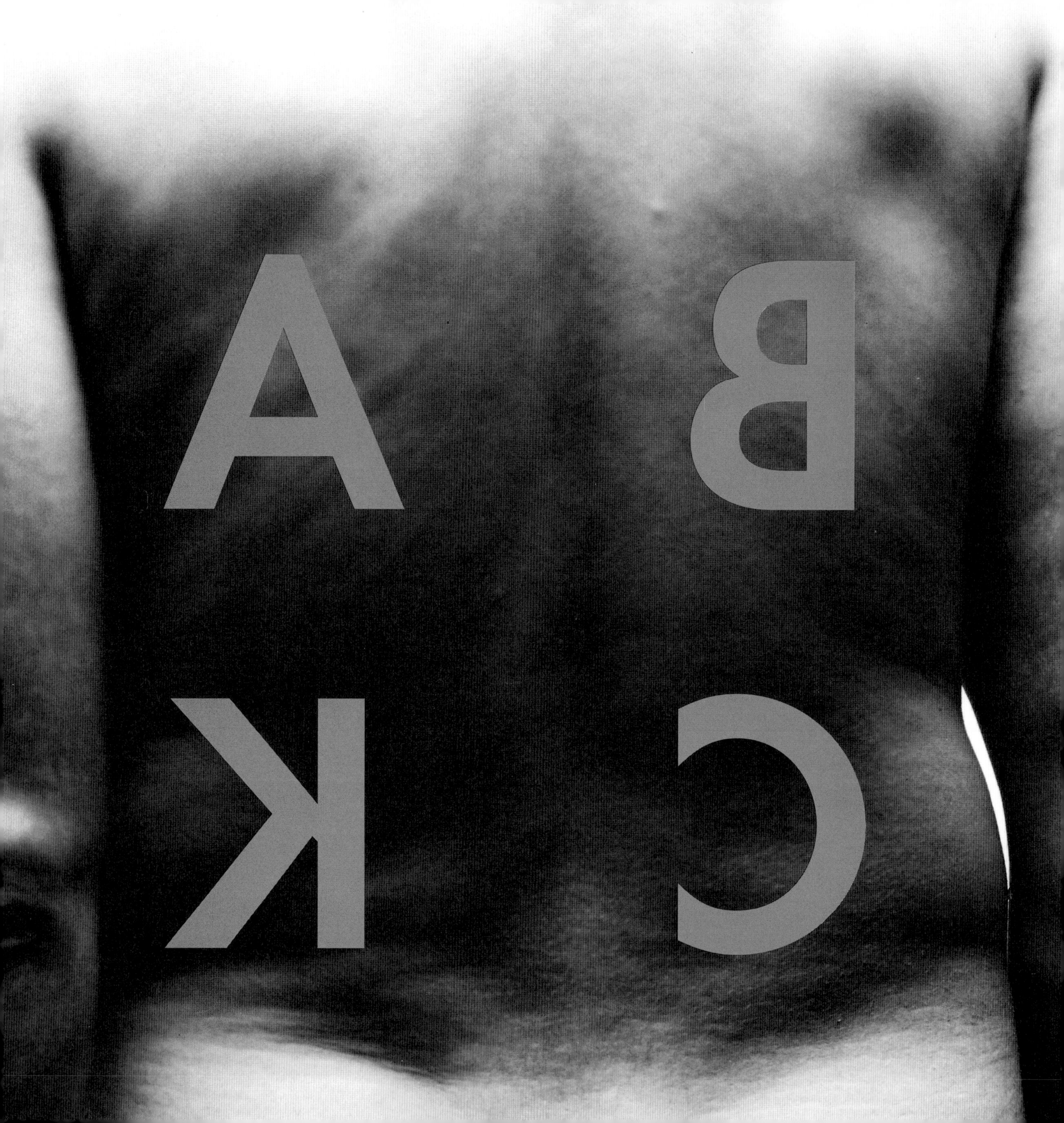
A
B
K
C

B A C K

THE SPINAL COLUMN HOLDS US ERECT. IT IS THE CENTER OF OUR STRENGTH, ENHANCING STABILITY, MOTION, AND FLEXIBILITY. THE SPINE consists of 24 joined bones, or vertebrae, layered in a slight S curve from the pelvis to the skull. Between the vertebrae are spongy disks that cushion the bones; openings in each vertebra form a protective channel for the spinal cord. Major nerves, connecting the spinal cord with other parts of the body, pass through spaces between the vertebrae and fill the muscles of the back with sensitivity. And anyone who's ever coughed up thousands of dollars for a chiropractor knows that the lower part of this column—the lumbar region—can be extremely sensitive. The lower back is one of the most vulnerable parts of our bodies. Disk problems account for only a small percentage of bad backs. The fault lies mostly in our muscles, which weaken with disuse, becoming more susceptible to strains.

MAINTENANCE: Backaches are the second leading cause of missed work in the U.S., after the common cold. Four out of five Americans will experience serious back pain at some point in their lives. **PREVENTION:** The best solution for back pain is prevention—don't wait until the pain becomes severe. Many problems may be alleviated by common sense: use an office seat with adequate support for the lower spine; do ten minutes of stretching, particularly on stressful days; learn to pick up heavy objects using the leg muscles, not the back muscles. People with desk jobs who try to transform themselves into weekend warriors are particularly prone to back problems: the muscles in the back need to be gradually exercised over time. **EXERCISE:** The key to a strong back is a strong stomach. Those who already have back problems need to consult a trainer or physical therapist to create an exercise program that will strengthen without strain.

[BACK *first aid—pages 207–208*]

M U S C L E S

THEY ENHANCE MOVEMENT—BOTH THE MOVEMENT THAT ALLOWS US TO ACT— voluntary muscle—and the movement that allows us to live—involuntary and cardiac muscle. With age, muscles lose their resilience and become less flexible. Muscle soreness was once thought to be caused by lactic acid. Lactic acid is the stuff that builds up in muscles with quick, heavy exertion such as weight lifting. Yet lactic acid is washed out of muscle tissue about 30 minutes after you stop exercising, and your muscles are still sore. Today, researchers think muscles get sore because of microscopic rips in the muscle tissue. The damage is apparently done not during the contracting phase of the exercise, but in the lengthening phase: in other words, not when you run up, but when you run down the hill.

MAINTENANCE: The best way to build or maintain muscles is through your favorite recreational exercise or weight training. **A NO-FRILLS OVERALL MUSCLE-BUILDING APPROACH / THREE TIMES A WEEK:** Three 30-minute sessions a week of aerobic exercise, such as running or cycling (or comparable, lighter exercise for about 45 minutes). Aerobic exercise is not so much for shaping the body as for keeping the heart in good working order. **WEIGHT TRAINING:** Begin with three 30-minute sessions, alternating upper-body and lower-body exercises (do not exercise the same set of muscles on consecutive days; muscles need time to heal). If possible, an investment in one or two sessions with a trainer to map out the best regimen for your body can speed things up. Obviously, the regimen will vary, depending on your goals. **STRETCHING:** The best time to stretch is after a workout, not before. Muscles do not turn to fat, but they do atrophy with lack of use. **SLOW DOWN:** Look for aerobic or calisthenics classes with slower music. Fast-paced music often means you're not getting the muscle extension you need for maintenance exercise.

[MUSCLES *first aid—page 208*]

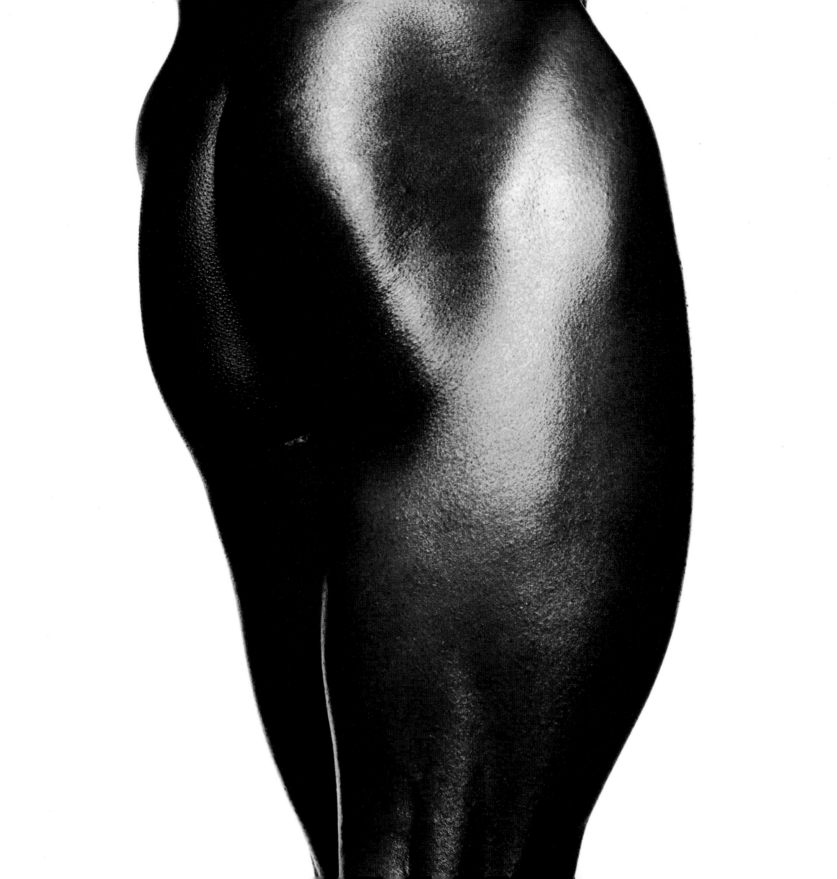

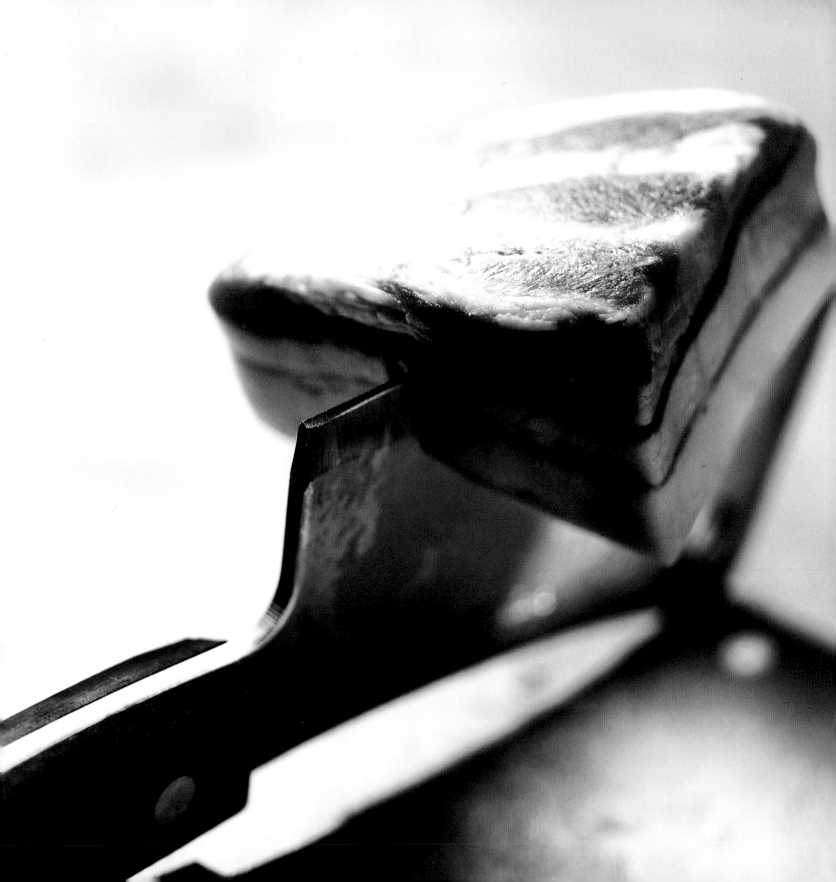

F A T

LITERATURE HAS GIVEN US DOZENS OF LOVABLE, CORPULENT ECCENTRICS: PICKWICK, FALSTAFF, MRS. CATHERINE MINGOTT. Fictional baddies tend to be scrawny, like Dickens's sepulchral Mr. Murdstone, or Shakespeare's "lean and hungry" Cassius. In our culture, obesity has taken on a moral stigma, despite the fact that it seems that a propensity for weight gain is genetic. Extreme thinness isn't recommended, since recent research shows that being too thin is linked with greater risk of early death than being slightly overweight. Being more than 20 percent above your ideal body weight does have health risks, from heart disease to diabetes, and for women, breast cancer.

The fat backlash (why a certain amount of fat is good)
We need a diet of about 10% fat for normal metabolic function.

Fat protects us from cold (ever notice how a man with a butt is a human hot-water bottle in bed?).

A woman needs some body fat to have children; without it, her menstrual cycle will stop.

Let's face it—fat fills up wrinkles and plump faces look younger.

When you're having a bad food day
Try to skip the butter on the bread, the oily salad dressing, the cream in the coffee, and the Häagen-Dazs nightcap. Eat one Yodel in a package of two.

Real world
Approximately 95% of people who attempt to lose weight by dieting alone fail. Exercise must be a part of any weight-maintenance program.

MAINTENANCE: The best protection against a lifetime of obesity is, unfortunately, out of your control: make sure you have slim parents who don't overfeed you as a child. After adolescence, the number of fat cells in a person's body remains constant over time (the only way to lessen the number of fat cells is by liposuction)—but those cells can expand or contract with alteration in eating habits and exercise. **WHY CUTTING CALORIES DOESN'T WORK:** When you restrict calories, the body goes on red alert. The body, knowing there is less fuel coming in, switches to "starvation mode" and begins doing everything possible to conserve energy. This is why nutritionists believe it becomes harder to lose weight after repeated dieting: our metabolisms get wise to us and simply slow down in anticipation of the next fasting period. In addition to causing mild fatigue and occasional light-headedness, reducing calorie intake forces the body to hold on to its fat supply with the tenacity of an aging diva clinging to the stage. It takes exercise to speed up the metabolism and force off the diva.

[FAT *first aid—page 208*]

LIPOSUCTION—RHYMES WITH "HYPO," ALTHOUGH WE PREFER TO THINK IT RHYMES WITH "HIPPO"—IS THE MOST COMMON FORM OF PLASTIC SURGERY IN THE U.S. MANY PEOPLE HAVE MULTIPLE LIPOSUCTION PROCEDURES. EIGHTY-SEVEN PERCENT OF ALL PATIENTS ARE WOMEN; 42 PERCENT OF THOSE WOMEN have fat removed from the thighs and hips. Most of the men have the procedure performed either on the stomach or to correct a condition known as gynecomastia (excess breast tissue). Liposuction works best on outer thighs, inner knees, buttocks, abdomen, and neck; it's iffier on inner legs and upper arms, where skin is thinner and less elastic. Liposuction is often combined with other surgeries: contouring a facelift, for example. Liposuction looks easy: you take what looks like a straw (called a cannula), insert it into the body, turn on a little suction pump (about one atmosphere of suction, a bit more than the best vacuum cleaner), and just sort of hoover away until the appropriate amount of fat, mixed with blood and other tissue, comes out. Up to two liters of fat (about four and a half pounds of flesh) can be safely removed from the body at any one time. Because liposuction is becoming increasingly common and safe, people tend to forget they're getting body tissue removed, not a new haircut. Liposuction is easy to do, but difficult to do well.

POSTOP: To reduce swelling and bruising, the patient wears a knees-to-waist surgical girdle for one to two months, and maybe more. **WARNING #1:** Girdles do not breathe. Do not plan to recuperate from this surgery in, say, August. **WARNING #2:** You can make love two weeks after surgery, although liposuction is definitely not conducive to romance. **POST-POSTOP:** The first week after surgery, you can walk; in the second and third weeks, you can swim; after the fourth and fifth weeks, you can take aerobics classes, dance, and bike. **WHAT YOU'RE NOT TOLD:** The need for continual fluid replenishment during surgery means that, for 12 hours after surgery, you must urinate about every 10 minutes, just at a time when—if you've had liposuction on your hips and thighs—sitting down is about as comfortable as swallowing molten lead. **WHAT ELSE YOU'RE NOT TOLD:** Liposuction aches for a much longer time than your doctor will admit to you. The soreness comes from lymph fluid trapped underneath the skin, which takes months to dissipate, and from the fact that the skin has been separated from the tissue structures underneath and takes a long time to reattach itself.

DANGERS: EXTREMELY RARE: Since 1982, approximately twelve people have died, some from complications resulting from anesthesia, and several from fat emboli caused by physicians who were too rough in dislodging fatty tissue. **LESS RARE:** If too much fat is removed, the result could be dimpling, waviness, or hanging skin—which can only be corrected by skin resectioning. **AVOIDING DANGER:** Check your doctor's credentials, and make sure he or she has operating privileges in a hospital with a good reputation. Additionally, ask to see some of his former patients in person. Pictures can, and do, lie. **WHO IT'S FOR:** Liposuction is for individuals with localized deposits of fat that no amount of exercise is going to eradicate. **WHO IT'S NOT FOR:** Liposuction is not recommended for those who are obese overall or lack skin elasticity—the skin must snap back to accommodate the fat loss. **THE FUTURE:** Some physicians believe liposuction will soon have uses beyond the cosmetic—for example, liposuction may be performed in stages for people suffering from diabetes or severe hypertension brought on by obesity, where weight loss has become a life-or-death issue.

"All this flat-belly
bullshit is killing the country."

JACK NICHOLSON

TU M MY

ALTHOUGH THE EXPANDING BELLY COMES SECOND ONLY TO THE RECEDING HAIRLINE IN THE PANTHEON OF MALE BODILY OBSESSIONS (OKAY, MAYBE THIRD), SOME WOMEN FIND A LITTLE AVOIRDUPOIS RATHER ENTICING. SOMETHING ABOUT A LOW CENTER OF GRAVITY MAKES THEM MORE STABLE in the saddle. Think Hell's Angels. Think corporate titans. Think cowboys (contrary to the Gary Cooper image, one rarely sees a real cowboy over 35 who's rangy). Even if you enjoy a mate shaped like a hot-water bottle, you shouldn't encourage them. For reasons that are still unclear, there's a correlation between stomach fat and heart disease.

MAINTENANCE: **AEROBIC:** When men burn fat with aerobic exercise, they lose it first in the abdomen. According to one study, older men who completed an aerobic exercise program dropped 20 percent of the fat from their midsection in six months. Also useful: cross-country skiing, stair climbing, and cycling. **CRUNCHES:** They don't get rid of fat, but crunches and other stomach exercises tighten and strengthen the muscles lying atop your stomach, which helps make the belly look smaller by altering posture. **SMOKING:** Smokers tend to accumulate fat on their bellies more than non-smokers; scientists speculate that smoking causes hormones to steer more fat to the waist. **DIET:** Alter your diet. Fat breeds fat.

OPTIONS: Love handles are to men what saddlebags are to women. Once those fat deposits land on your body, they're extremely difficult to shoo away by conventional means. **LIPOSUCTION—"TUMMY TUCK":** With a stomach liposuction, a tiny little incision is made in the stomach and a strawlike device is inserted to suck away the fat. The tummy tuck is usually reserved for those who have gained and then lost a large amount of weight, and whose stomach is stretched and sagging; here, excess skin is removed and the area is restructured to ensure your belly button does not end up somewhere around your shoulders. Vacuuming your middle may be an immediate answer but aerobics is forever.

John Thomas Sausage
Wee Willie The Pickle.
Boner Woody Salami
Peter Lead-Pipe Wanker
Schlong Stick Piece Rod
Joint Snake Dong Prick
Dork Privates Cock Injector
Weener Throbbing Beef
Long-John One-Eyed
Trouser Snake Dick
The Little Man
Ding-a-Ling Mr. Jones
The General Lemon
Licorice-Stick Shaft
Noodle Love-Muscle
Shaking Hands With
the President

"A MAN FALLS IN LOVE THROUGH HIS EYES; A WOMAN, THROUGH HER EARS," A WAG ONCE OBSERVED. WHEN a man sees something arousing, his brain sends signals to shut off the outflow of blood in the penis. The blood is trapped; the penis rises purplish and stiff. After continued

Average male "inch"

Average penis size
5 to 7 inches

Minimum size necessary to join Hung Jury, a California dating service that matches men with women who like their dates well hung
8 inches

MAINTENANCE: **POTENCY AND AGING:** To say a man's sexual performance peaks at 18 is true, but only if you equate "performance" with quantity of erections—which most women, at least, do not do. Their erections may be bit less firm and orgasm may take longer, but most men are capable of enjoying sex well into their nineties. **PROSTATE HEALTH:** The prostate is a gland about the size of a walnut that produces seminal fluid during ejaculation. The urethra

P E N I S

friction, the testicles are pulled closer to the body, and orgasm, muscular contractions that propel semen out of the penis, occurs. After an orgasm, men either sleep, eat a sandwich, or write bad poetry.

Attention Hung Jury rejects
A smaller penis will increase more in size during an erection than a large one.

passes through the prostate—when it enlarges, common in men over 55, the urethra is narrowed and the man has difficulty urinating. Men over 50 should have their prostates examined annually; a simple blood test can tell whether there's an increase in the level of cancer-related antigens. Prostate cancer is one of the most frequent cancers among men.

"All that you suspect about women's friendships is true. We talk about dick size."

CYNTHIA HEIMEL

[PENIS *first aid—pages 208–209*]

V   A   G

THE ROMAN PHILOSOPHER LUCRETIUS LIKED TO COUNSEL WIVES

not to move during intercourse, since "a woman prevents and battles pregnancy because if

in her joy she answers the man's lovemaking with her buttocks, and her soft breasts billow for-

ward and back; for she diverts the ploughshare out of the furrow and makes the seed miss its

mark." And so goes the para-

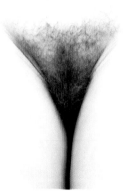

dox of a woman's sexuality: we

are built for enjoyment, but

watch out if you're having too

much fun. Women generally

need more tactile stimulation

than men to become aroused;

a picture (even one of Mel

Gibson) just doesn't do it. With kissing and caressing, the woman's breathing becomes more

rapid, and her heart beats quickly; the vagina becomes moist; the clitoris swells and becomes

engorged; the vagina lengthens and distends during the "plateau" phase of excitement; and,

eventually, the body shudders with orgasm 10 to 15 contractions at .8-second intervals, to be exact.

I N A

MAINTENANCE: Our culture teaches us that aging is synonymous with loss of sexual desirability and sexual desire. More and more research shows that sex drive in women is more affected by emotional factors—stress, concern about appearance, distraction from children—than physical ones. In fact, women's sexual peak arrives much later than man's, in the late thirties to mid-forties. There can be a change in, but not a loss of, sexual feeling with the advent of menopause. **AVOIDING VAGINAL MUSCLE FLACCIDITY:** There is some truth in the phrase "Use it or lose it." Regular sex is useful in maintaining the muscle condition of the vagina. And muscle condition can also be maintained by doing kegel exercises: Simply tightening and relaxing the "kegels" or muscles surrounding the vagina (the same ones that control urinary flow) can help make sex more enjoyable for both men and women. **DEALING WITH PMS:** The biggest culprits of the water retention that accompanies PMS are fluid-retainers such as salt and caffeine. Cutting down on them may make all the difference between mild swelling and the beached-whale look—making it safe to fall asleep on the beach again. Daily doses of B vitamins and folic acid are also reported to reduce irritability and cramping. **MINIMIZING THE SYMPTOMS OF MENOPAUSE:** You may be one of the lucky ones who have virtually none of the classic symptoms of menopause: hot flashes, night sweats and insomnia, mood swings, increased hairiness, vaginal dryness during intercourse (all are caused, in one way or another, by the diminishing level of estrogen in the body). On the other hand, estrogen-replacement therapy is saving millions of women from an otherwise uncomfortable "change of life." Unfortunately, many women are cavalier about estrogen-replacement therapy: there are risks (women with a history of breast cancer in the family should probably avoid it). Anyone considering this option should be thoroughly evaluated by her physician.

[VAGINA *first aid—pages 209–10*]

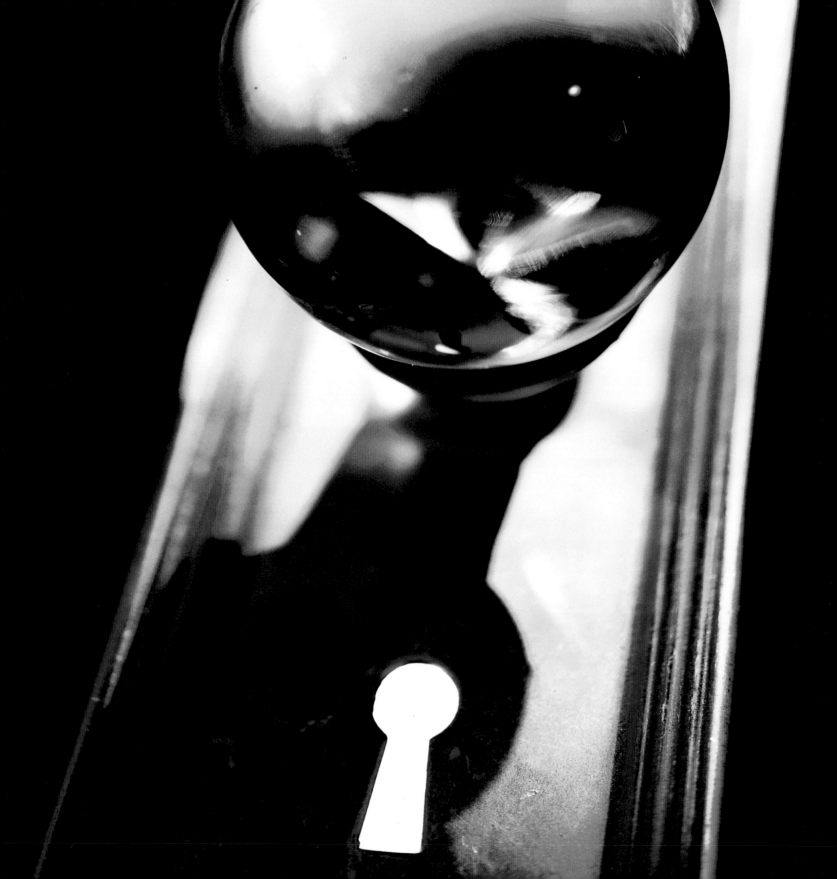

L U S T

WHEN DID IT FIRST STRIKE? WHILE YOU WERE SNOOPING AROUND YOUR PARENTS' BEDROOM AND FOUND THEIR COLLECTION of X-rated videos? The first time you read *Portnoy's Complaint,* and found yourself skipping to the "good parts"? Lust first necessitates a recognition of and fascination with the Other. It combines the burning desire for familiarity with the necessity of mystery. Once it's experienced, we are never the same. Most women's desire level acts as a natural contraceptive: we

Tell us something we didn't know

When psychologists at Arizona State University questioned 327 college students about their criteria for marriage and steady dating, both men and women sought similar qualities: intelligence, social status, attractiveness. But for one-night stands, women maintained their standards while men acted "like other mammals— undiscriminating," said one researcher. Men were willing to overlook minor considerations like intelligence and personality.

are most amorous just after and just before our periods (the time when we're least likely to get pregnant) and many of us become more interested in shopping at about the same time we ovulate. Whereas most women regard physical intimacy as the outgrowth of emotional intimacy, many men find emotional intimacy through sex; in fact, sex may be man's primary way of expressing closeness. Of course, sex may also be a man's way of expressing nothing more than pleasure, or the relief of tension.

"Masturbation is the thinking man's television."

CHRISTOPHER HAMPTON

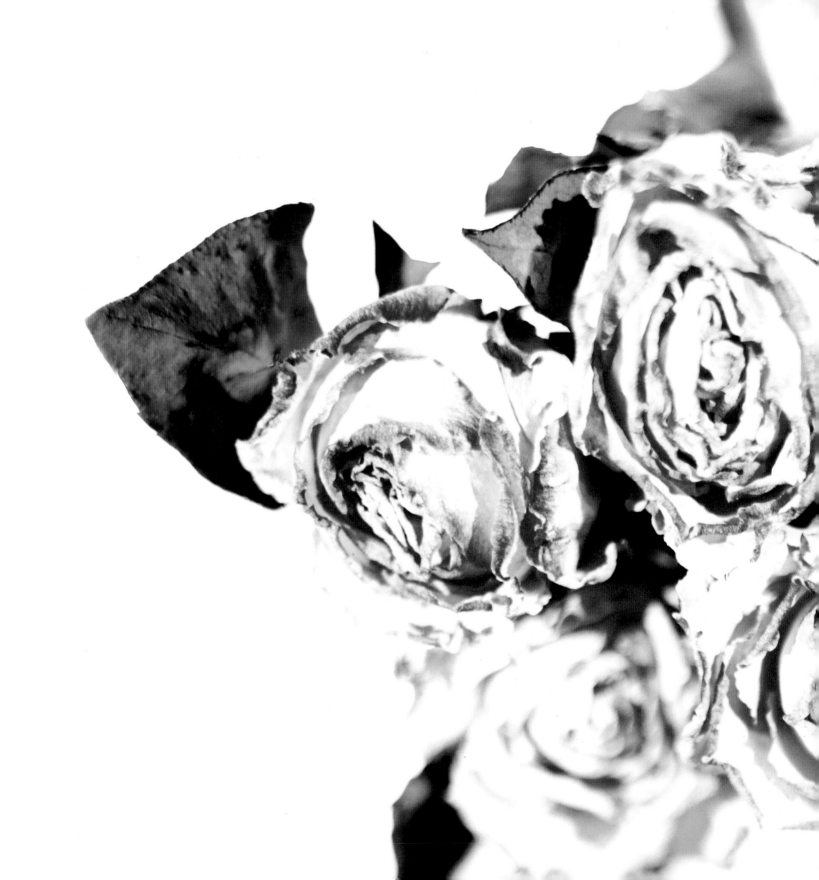

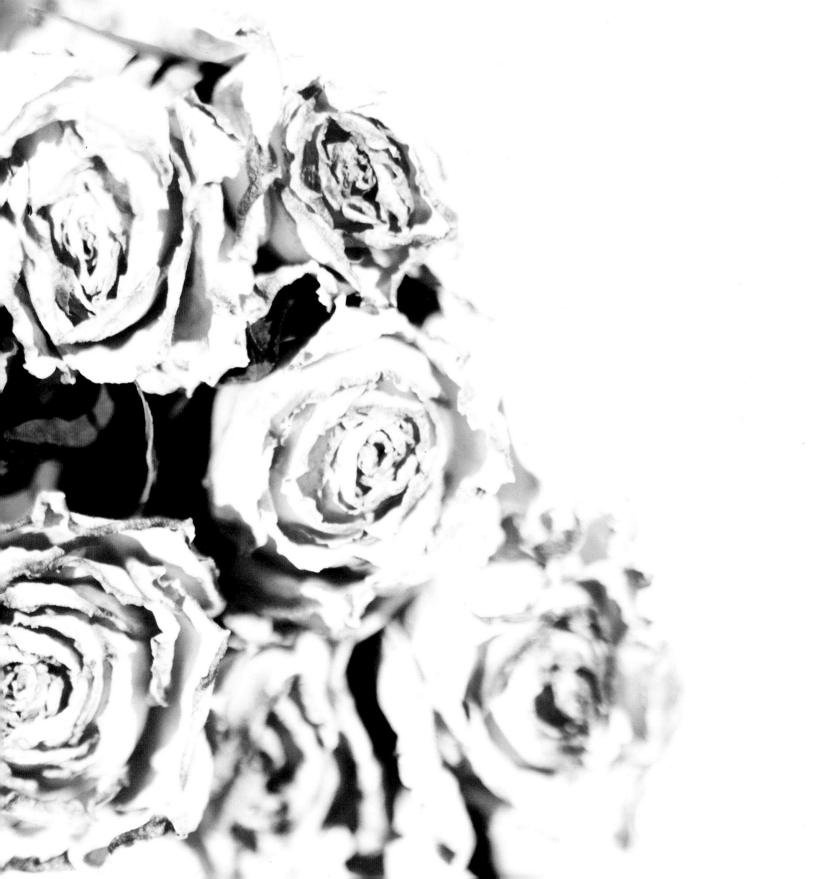

S E X

THERE'S NO SUCH THING AS "TOO MUCH MASTURBATION"; IN FACT, MASTURBATION IS A NECESSITY IN FIGURING OUT what our bodies want and conveying that information to a partner. With age, masturbation becomes more important—with or without partners. For a woman, it increases lubrication for those times we are with a partner. Emotionally, for both sexes, well, Woody Allen was right after all: sex is best with someone you love.

Number of Americans who masturbate

160,512,000

Number of Americans who have experienced oral sex

155,040,000

Sadomasochistic sex

10,944,000

The average American woman has sexual intercourse

2,879 times

The average American male

3,778 times

The average American has 4,438 orgasms

Not so impressive, when you consider we live an average of 75 years, or 27,375 days.

MAINTENANCE: **ORGASM:** Is there a difference between what men feel and women feel during orgasm? We'll never know for sure. **G-WHIZ:** The vagina itself is not filled with erectile nerve tissue and therefore, according to Masters and Johnson, there is no such thing as vaginal orgasm. But there is an area inside the front wall of the vagina, called the G-spot, which many women claim can be stimulated to orgasm. The G-spot orgasm is in some cases even more intense than a clitoral orgasm. Researchers are unsure whether all women have a G-spot. **GREAT SEX:** Unfortunately, we are a performance-driven society, and sexual comparison can be alienating and self-defeating. As the joke goes, the greatest sex is the last sex you had.

"In my sex fantasy, nobody ever loves me for my mind."

NORA EPHRON

[SEX *first aid—page 210*]

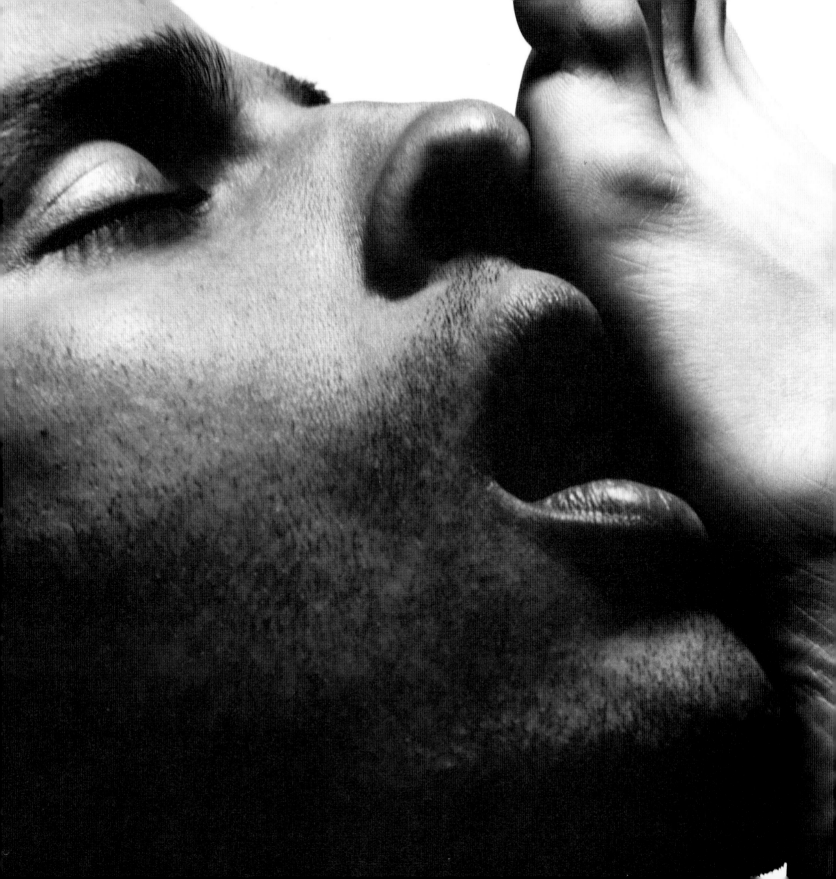

"I'd be a **dog-faced liar** if I told you that I don't enjoy slithering around in those **pretty panties** and bras that I can now order from the catalogs and actually fit into and look fabulous in. If putting on the black thigh-high stockings, push-up bra, and **black spiked heels**—just before the dress goes on—and seeing my husband's jaw drop to the ground and loving every moment of it are rooted in some **warped** sexual representation…then so be it. It's big fun parading around in those sexy things, and for all the **feminists** of the world reading this book, I am not doing it for him. I'm **doing it for me.**"

The former 260-pound housewife-turned-infomercial-queen has developed a fitness/wellness program called "Stop the Insanity!" based on her own self-developed journey to fitness. Her no-nonsense, common-sense approach comes from painful personal experience with failed dieting, a fitness industry geared to the already fit, and a medical/nutrition establishment slow to endorse the importance of low-fat, high-quality foods. Emphasizing the goal as getting lean, strong, and healthy (although her goal was to look better than her ex-husband's girlfriend), the program boils down to EAT (low-fat, quality food in unlimited quantity; food is fuel), MOVE (get your heart rate up for 30 minutes every day), and BREATHE (fat burns in oxygen). That's it. Powter also tells politically incorrect tales on herself, both wrathful and victorious. She may be of the moment but her information is timeless.

SUSAN POWTER

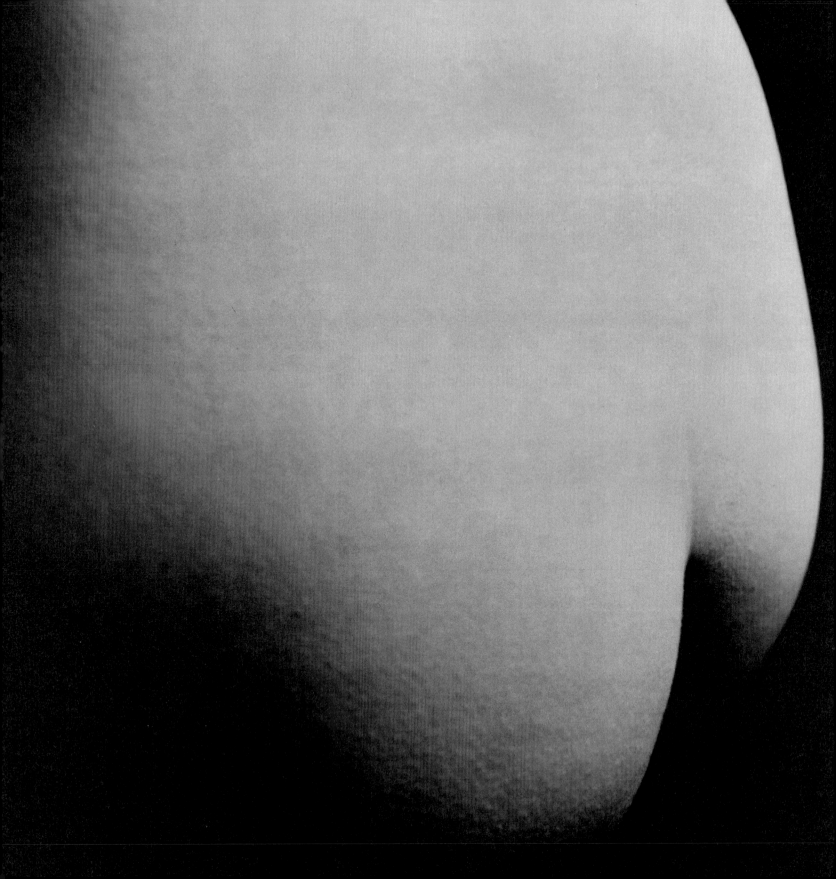

BUTTOCKS

MALE APPRECIATION OF THE FEMALE POSTERIOR IS RECIPROCAL: IN STUDY AFTER STUDY, WOMEN CITE BUTTOCKS AS ONE OF THE FIRST PARTS of the body they notice on a man, usually right after eyes. A recent series of ads in Japan designed to interest women in baseball featured close-ups of the players' bottoms. Interestingly, the buttocks are one part of the human body where men's taste is more catholic than women's: women prefer small and hard, while men's taste runs the gamut from boyish and tight to expansive, soft, and squeezable. Men interested in women's derrieres consider themselves connoisseurs of shape, proportion, and wiggle-quotient. Breast-men, with their emphasis on mere size, are vulgarians by comparison. Interestingly, though, the buttocks as an erogenous zone are an area of deeper ambivalence than breasts: they are sexual, but, as they involve excretory functions, they are also considered dirty. Still, just as the '50s were the decade of the breast, this may be the decade of the buttock. Once again fashion follows fetish: the athletic emphasis of today has obviously shaped and focused more than the biceps and thighs in America's consciousness.

MAINTENANCE: Glutes are among our largest muscles; they atrophy with age. The result is sagging and spreading. Strong gluteal muscles facilitate leg motion and help in lifting and propulsion. Without strong glutes, it's easier to injure your lower back muscles disproportionately with lifting. Your buttocks' width is not entirely under your control, but their strength and firmness are. **GOOD RECREATIONAL SPORTS:** In-line skating, cross-country skiing, racket sports. **EXERCISES:** Leg lunges; leg lifts; lying on back, contracting and relaxing buttocks. Repeat desired exercise three times a week, with a day of rest in between. Start with one set of 10 to 12 repetitions, aiming for three sets of 15 to 20.

[BUTTOCKS *first aid—page 210*]

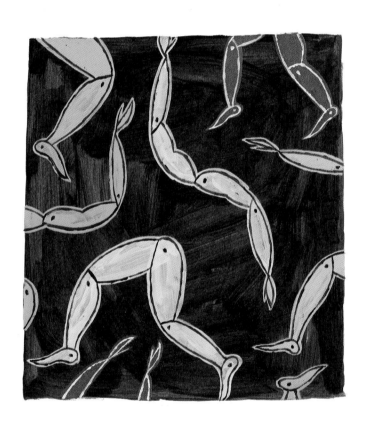

LIMBS

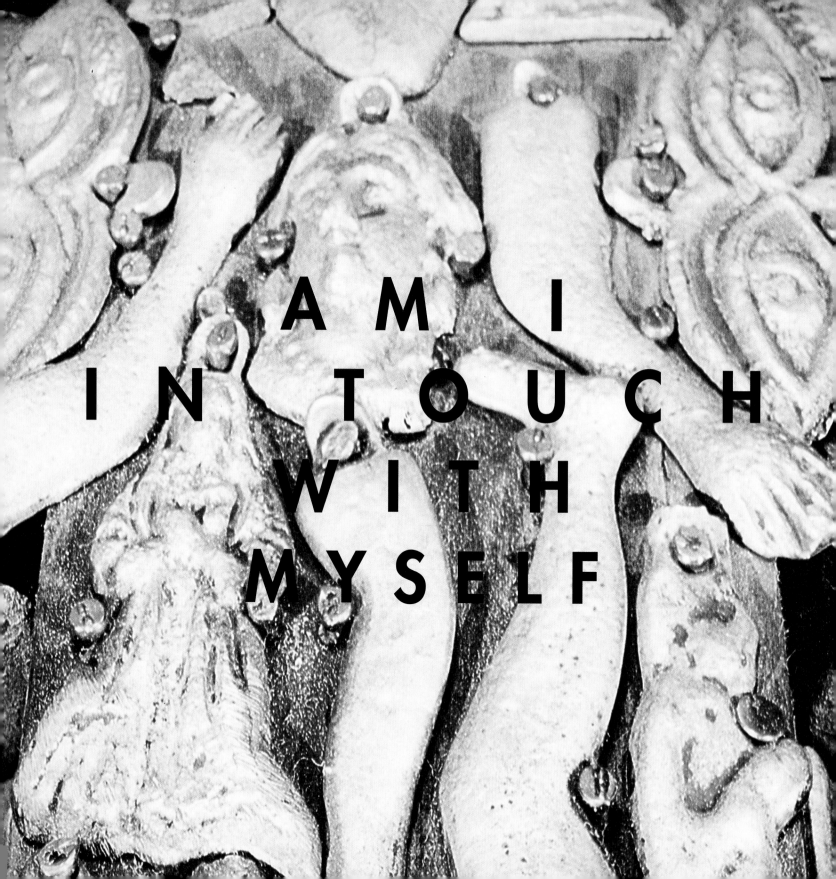

It's very simple: our limbs give us the gift of touch, and if human beings didn't love to touch, the species would have died off long ago. Touch is not only the most primitive of our senses, but perhaps the most important to our early development. When a baby is born, it is at first swaddled: holding his limbs close to his body seems to provide a sense of security. Even if a baby's ability to touch is in this way monitored, it is critical for the baby to be touched by others: in fact, repeated studies have found that babies who are regularly massaged gain weight 50 percent more quickly than unmassaged babies, and at the age of 6 months, the massaged babies did better on tests of mental and motor ability. As much as sight and sound, touch orients us in our worlds. The touch of a lover, too, becomes as deeply imprinted in our minds as his face or voice. Watch an elderly couple holding hands. Their faces may be sagging and their voices cracked; but that touch is the same touch they gave each other as ardent 20-year-olds. And they know it.

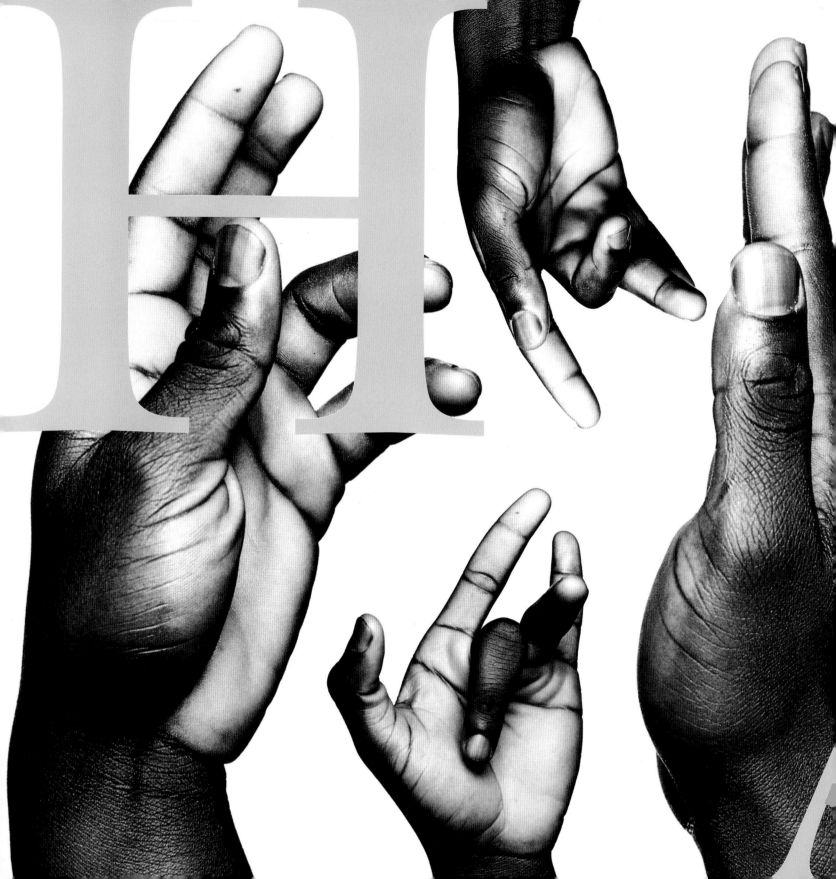

"REACH OUT AND TOUCH SOMEONE": IN THAT ONE MEMORABLE LINE, AT&T MANAGED TO EQUATE THE POWER OF TECHNOLOGY WITH THE POWER OF HUMAN CONTACT. IT IS A GREAT POWER—SO MUCH SO THAT THE HANDSHAKE, WHICH WAS ONCE A way for two warriors to show they had no concealed weapons, has become the universal Western gesture for expressing good faith. The importance of touch goes infinitely beyond the sexual; it is the Spackle which we use to smooth daily social transactions. For example, in an experiment in Oxford, Mississippi, waitresses were told to selectively touch some diners lightly on the hand or shoulder. Those customers who were touched didn't necessarily rate the food or restaurant higher, but they consistently gave better tips to the waitresses. The hand is one of our most simple and direct tools of communication.

MAINTENANCE: Hand shape, of course, is predetermined, but two things can be done in the name of upkeep. **WASHING:** A good reason to wash your hands several times a day is to cut down on the number of colds you get during the year. The cold virus is airborne, and you can also catch it from touching surfaces on which someone with a cold has breathed or sneezed. Washing your hands helps to remove the virus. **A SIMPLE PLEASURE:** Rubbing moisturizer on your hands not only alleviates dryness and keeps skin silky but also gives you a chance to massage key pressure points and refresh nerve endings.

[HANDS *first aid—pages 210–11*]

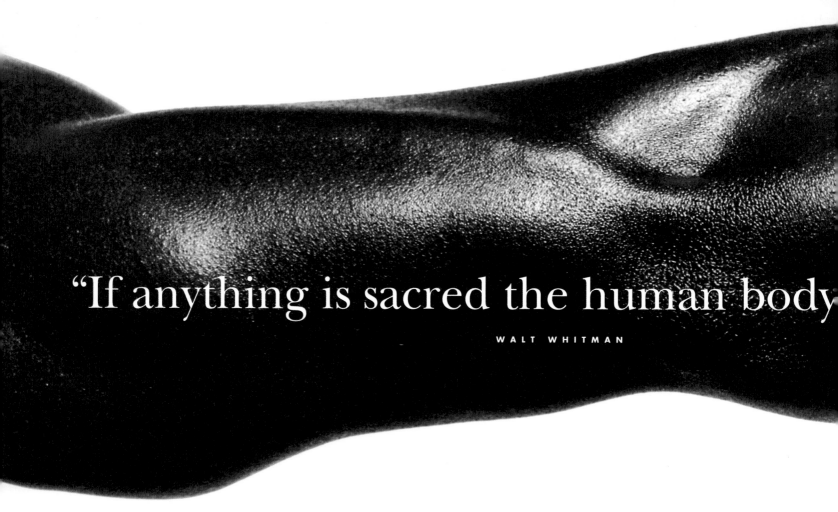

"If anything is sacred the human body

WALT WHITMAN

IN RECENT YEARS THERE HAS BEEN A DRASTIC CHANGE IN PEOPLE'S NOTIONS OF FEMALE BEAUTY WHERE ARMS ARE CONCERNED. A BEAUTIFUL FEMALE ARM WAS THIN BUT SOFT, STRONG ENOUGH TO CRADLE A BABY BUT STILL WEAK ENOUGH TO REQUIRE HELP BRINGING IN THE GROCERIES. A WOMAN WITH strong, well-defined arm muscles was repulsive, vaguely threatening, almost perverse; today, that same arm is the ideal. Arms are one of the few body parts that men are more obsessive about than women are. Bulging biceps are the most visible symbol of a man's strength and masculinity; you can go to any gym and see men with sticklike legs and rotund bellies who nevertheless spend hours creating arms a highland gorilla would be proud of.

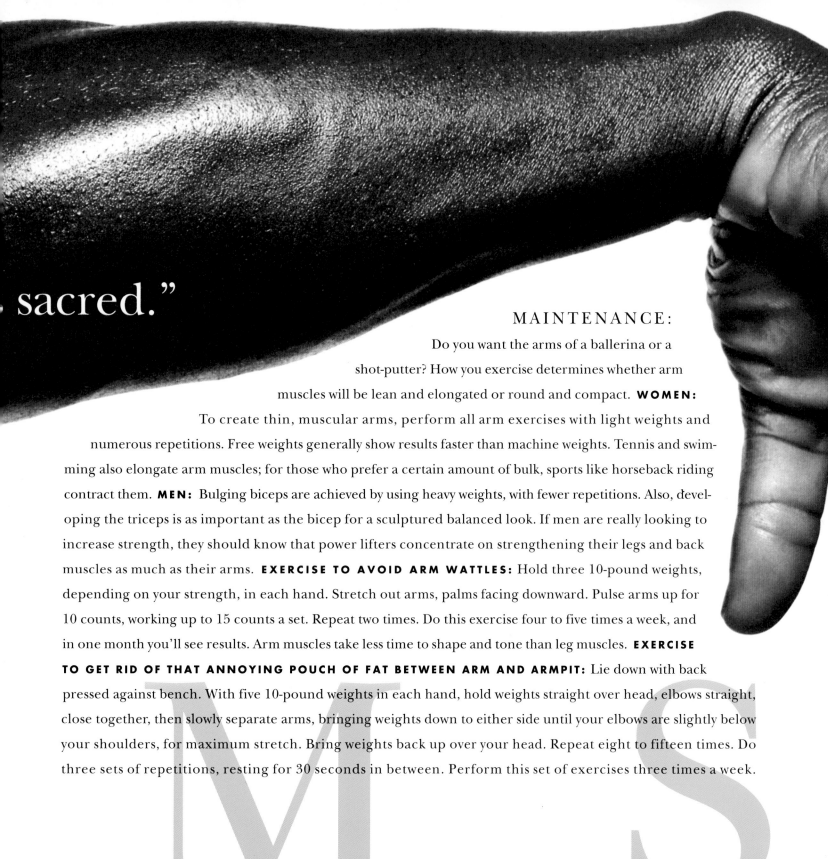

sacred."

MAINTENANCE:

Do you want the arms of a ballerina or a shot-putter? How you exercise determines whether arm muscles will be lean and elongated or round and compact. **WOMEN:** To create thin, muscular arms, perform all arm exercises with light weights and numerous repetitions. Free weights generally show results faster than machine weights. Tennis and swimming also elongate arm muscles; for those who prefer a certain amount of bulk, sports like horseback riding contract them. **MEN:** Bulging biceps are achieved by using heavy weights, with fewer repetitions. Also, developing the triceps is as important as the bicep for a sculptured balanced look. If men are really looking to increase strength, they should know that power lifters concentrate on strengthening their legs and back muscles as much as their arms. **EXERCISE TO AVOID ARM WATTLES:** Hold three 10-pound weights, depending on your strength, in each hand. Stretch out arms, palms facing downward. Pulse arms up for 10 counts, working up to 15 counts a set. Repeat two times. Do this exercise four to five times a week, and in one month you'll see results. Arm muscles take less time to shape and tone than leg muscles. **EXERCISE TO GET RID OF THAT ANNOYING POUCH OF FAT BETWEEN ARM AND ARMPIT:** Lie down with back pressed against bench. With five 10-pound weights in each hand, hold weights straight over head, elbows straight, close together, then slowly separate arms, bringing weights down to either side until your elbows are slightly below your shoulders, for maximum stretch. Bring weights back up over your head. Repeat eight to fifteen times. Do three sets of repetitions, resting for 30 seconds in between. Perform this set of exercises three times a week.

F I N G E R N A I L S

A HANDSHAKE IS GENERALLY THE FIRST SENSUAL EXPERIENCE WE HAVE WITH ANOTHER PERSON, AND ONE OF THE FIRST THINGS WE NOTICE IS HIS OR HER NAILS. ARE THEY LONG? SHORT? BITTEN TO THE QUICK? COLORLESS POLISH? OR COLOR—AND HOW MUCH COLOR? NO POLISH AT ALL IS also a statement. Iconographically, nails are a sign of both female power and female helplessness: the power of feminine eros married to the vulnerability of a woman who, as Susan Brownmiller quips, can no longer make a fist. Women have been staining their fingernails with color derived from plants since Egyptian times; the color was thought to attract men and repel evil spirits. Until the 1920s, fashionable women in America would have their nails buffed with a rose powder. Then nail enamels came on the scene, a serendipitous use of what was originally developed as automobile paint.

MAINTENANCE: The well-groomed hand has been a mark of wealth and leisure—a sign, as Susan Brownmiller writes in *Femininity*, that "manual labor lies whimsically beyond its reach." **WHAT THEY ARE:** Nails, skin, and hair are related, each being made of a protein called keratin. Nails are highly porous. **DRY NAILS:** Nails lose moisture at a rate hundreds of times greater than skin. For dry nails, massage moisturizers into the nail's growth center, directly under the cuticle.

OPTIONS: Don't make them too interesting. They're nails, and they're most appealing when form and function are balanced. A healthy set of fingernails, groomed to a modest half-inch long (or less), with slightly rounded tips, and polished, if at all, with pale or clear lacquer, can go anywhere, with anything. MEN: With the growth of the hair salon for men, the manicure has become more common. Say no to clear polish, however; there's such a thing as being too groomed.

[NAILS *first aid—page 211*]

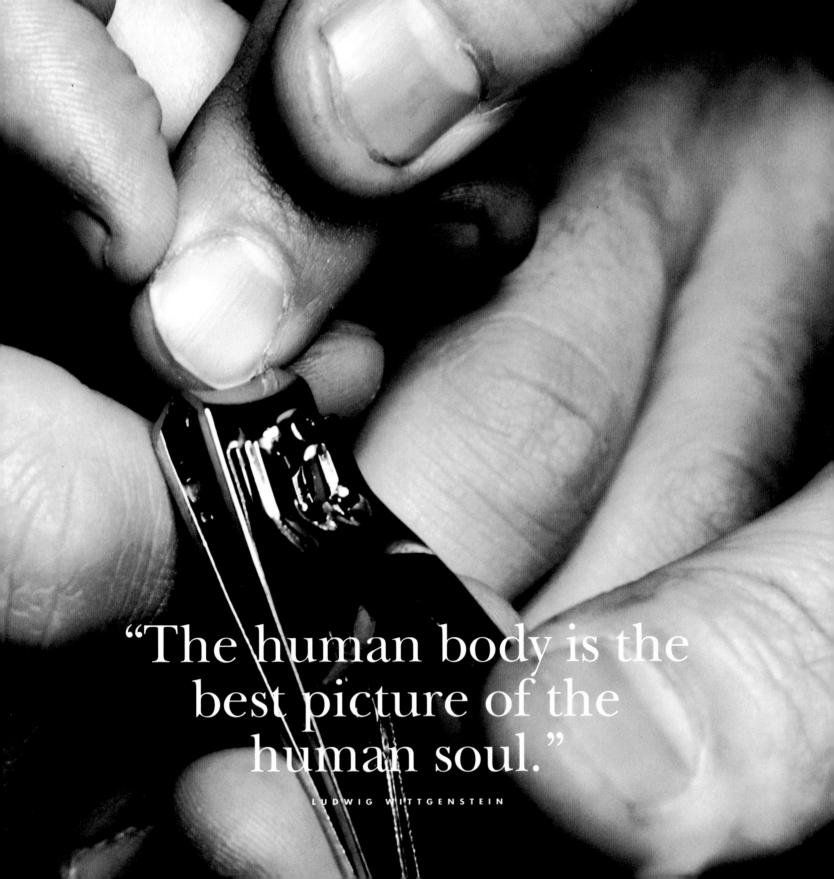

"The human body is the best picture of the human soul."

LUDWIG WITTGENSTEIN

L   E

OUR EXPERIENCE WITH LEGS BEGINS AT MOTHER'S KNEE:

WE FIRST USE HER LEGS TO HIDE FROM SCARY AUNT SADIE WITH

THE FAKE EYELASHES, WHO'S JUST DYING FOR A KISS. LATER, LEGS

BECOME QUITE LITERALLY A MEANS OF ESCAPE, AND LATER STILL A SEXUAL

object. In fact, some sex therapists even speculate that so-called leg   ose

who find legs particularly sexy—had mothers who tended   pick them up and

hug them to her breast when they were upset. Consequently, they clung to

her legs, and this became the first part of the female body   eroticized.

G S

MAINTENANCE: If you were not blessed from birth with legs like Julia Roberts, there's still hope.

CELLULITE: Cellulite is not water or "toxins" trapped beneath the skin's surface. It is, quite simply, fat. The way fat is distributed under the skin accounts for whether it's lumpy or not: some very heavy women have no cellulite at all, and some slim women still have "cottage-cheese" thighs. Men rarely have it, because their fat cells are arranged differently: whereas women tend to have fat cells that protrude outward when they gain weight, male fat cells form a horizontal, net

GETTING RID OF IT: Scientists are able to create babies in test tubes, but so far nobody has been able to come up with a plan for eradicating cellulite. Even liposuction, which removes fat cells, cannot change the way fat is distributed under the skin. Regular leg-toning exercises are the best—indeed, the only—way to minimize cellulite accumulation. **BEST EXERCISE:** Leg lunges. Stand in "fencing" position, lunging forward while placing your weight first on the right leg, then the left. Start with 20 lunges on each leg; work up to three sets of 20 lunges a day, or at least every other day.

[LEGS *first aid—page 212*]

F E

IT'S ODD TO CONSIDER THE FOOT AS AN OBJECT OF VENERATION. IT'S NEITHER GRACEFUL NOR CHARMING, AND IF NOT PROPERLY TENDED, IT SMELLS LIKE NOTHING ELSE ON THIS PLANET. YET AT ONE POINT IN CHINESE HISTORY (ABOUT 1000 A.D.), A TINY FOOT WAS THE SYMBOL OF BEAUTY, and normal-sized feet a symbol of shame. To ensure their daughters' desirability, mothers would mutilate them by binding their feet, thus compressing the bones and rendering them excruciatingly painful to walk on, if not gangrenous. Foot-binding was thought to alter the vagina, giving a man vastly more pleasure. At this time, artists could paint the raciest nudes, but the models' feet could never be shown uncovered. Even today, foot worship is among the most common fetishes. The foot is one of the switchboard areas for the nervous system. From tickling to acupressure, this sometimes callused surface is amazingly sensitive.

"Only two rules really count: never never miss an opportunity

E   T

MAINTENANCE: Here's a few tips for putting your best foot forward. **AVOIDING ATHLETE'S FOOT:** You wouldn't wear the same underwear seven days in a row, but many of us think nothing of wearing the same shoes daily. Shoes need a chance to dry out before they're worn again. If they don't, you increase the chance of contracting athlete's foot, a form of fungus which loves warm, moist places. **AVOIDING ACHING FEET:** Soaking works. Try dipping feet in a pot of barley or millet—two cups of grain to eight cups of water. Cook the barley on the stove until it's mushy; wait for it to cool, and plunge your feet in for about half an hour. Rinse with cold water and rub with rough towel. **AVOIDING SMELLY FEET:** Wash feet often, change socks every day, use charcoal shoe liners, and if all else fails, see a physician—there may be an underlying medical problem. **FOR CALLUSED FEET:** This is what petroleum jelly does best. Rub it into feet and put on a pair of socks. Wake up the next morning and feel the difference.

miss an opportunity to relieve yourself; to rest your feet." DUKE OF WINDSOR.

[FEET *first aid—page 212*]

WOULD SARAH, THE DUCHESS OF WINDSOR, HAVE CAUSED SUCH A STIR IF A NOSY PHOTOGRAPHER HAD CAUGHT HER COMPANION KISSING HER LIPS INSTEAD OF HER TOES? THE ROYAL TOE-SUCKING incident hit a bit too close to home: millions of people imagined themselves caught in this tiny act of excruciating intimacy, and squirmed. They're our favorite little piggies.

T O

MAINTENANCE: **AVOIDING CORNS AND CALLUSES:** These thickened and hardened patches of dead skin cells result from constant rubbing of a part of the foot against the shoe. Key to avoiding them: Get shoes that fit. This may seem obvious, but every one of us, at one time or another, has bought a pair of shoes a size too small because—well, we were foolish. **CURING:** Corns and calluses can be rubbed away with a pumice stone after a warm-water soak. Various over-the-counter medications are also available to soften and remove them. **AVOIDING BUNIONS:** These bony bumps on the side of the big toe typically develop when the big toe angles toward the other toes instead of pointing straight ahead, and the large bone at the base of the toe juts outward. Women develop bunions about ten times as often as men, probably because they force their feet into narrow, pointy, high-heeled shoes. And the prevalence of bunions increases with age, both because older people are more likely to have arthritis-related deformities and because their feet have gotten bigger while they think their shoe size remains the same. Avoiding them means wearing shoes that are wide enough, or protecting the protruding toe with a doughnut-shaped pad. **CURING:** Once a bunion has formed, it should only be treated by a podiatrist. **AVOIDING INGROWN TOENAILS:** Too-tight shoes, fungal infections, odd toe structures, injuries, pounding during aerobic exercise, and, especially, faulty toenail trimming can all cause toenails to become ingrown. Make sure toenails are cut with a toenail clipper—not scissors—straight across the toe—not curved, and not too short. **CURING:** If it's a really stubborn case, visit a podiatrist. But sometimes you can solve the problem yourself. First, soften the nail by soaking it in warm, soapy water. After drying it thoroughly, remove the dead skin and other yucky stuff from underneath the nail using an orangewood stick. Insert a wisp of sterile cotton in the nail groove, using your finger or the stick. Put a drop of antiseptic (such as Betadine solution) on the cotton, and wrap the toe with gauze and tape. Let the nail grow beyond the tip of the toe. Change the cotton when needed. **CURE FOR STUBBED TOE:** Rub toe very vigorously, literally inundating the skin's touch sensors with so much tactile information for the brain that the pain will subside in mass confusion.

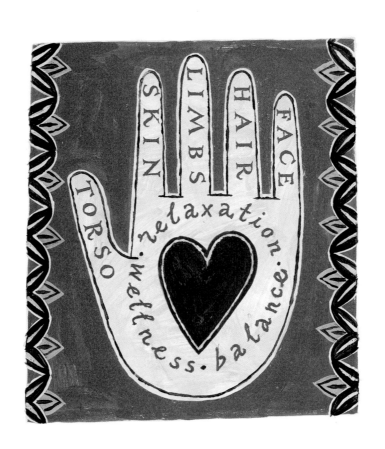

WHOLENESS

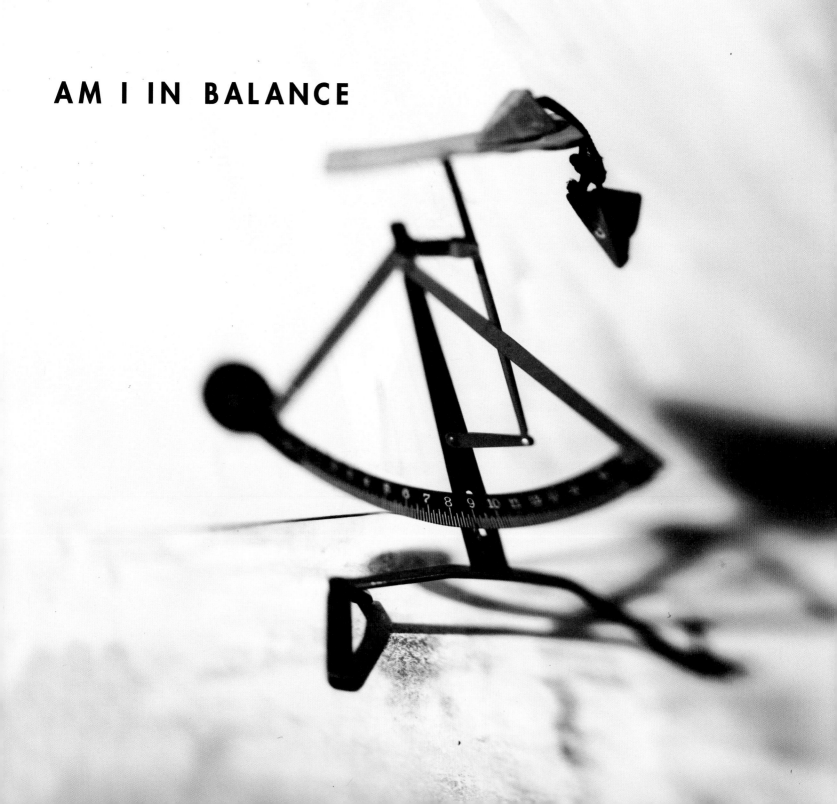

AM I IN BALANCE

This book has been about the physical: how to look your best, and how to keep yourself healthy and vibrant over the long haul. It's also about making choices—health and appearance are an obligation to no one but yourself. Still, we've only been talking about half the equation. Perfect teeth and shiny hair do not constitute beauty, although they help. It's a truism, but nonetheless a powerful one, that our inner life—and what we do to benefit it—shines through in our outward appearance. The mind matters.

STRESS

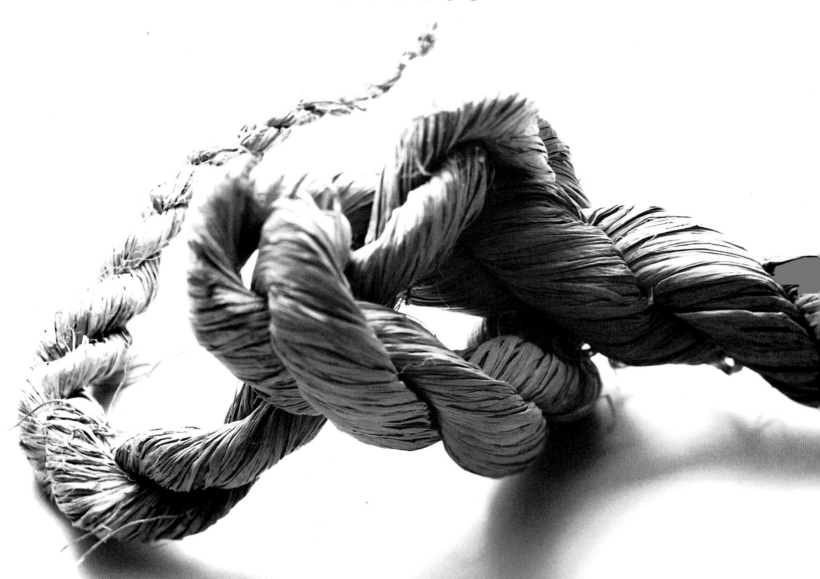

"I read this article, it said the typical symptoms of stress are eating
too much, smoking too much, impulse buying, and driving too fast.
Are they kidding? This is my idea of a great day!"

MONICA PIPER

ASKED RECENTLY HOW SHE DEALS WITH THE DAY-TO-DAY CRAZINESS OF HER WORK, A FAMOUS HOLLYWOOD AGENT REPORTEDLY REPLIED: "I'M AN OLD-FASHIONED GAL: I BELIEVE IN ANALYSIS AND PROZAC." FORTUNATELY, MANY OF US WITH EQUALLY FRENETIC LIVES ARE finding other alternatives. If we want to keep our health, not to mention our sanity, we must. Stress accounts for a formidable range of ailments, from back pain and neck pain to tension headaches, irritable bowel syndrome, teeth grinding, and even infertility. An Ohio State University College of Medicine study showed medical students exhibited weakened immune responses during exam period. Scientists have also found evidence that the immune responses of happily married couples break down after an argument. Their conclusion? Close personal relationships and self-disclosure seem to enhance health. The key to coping with stress is learning how not to be a victim and learning how to confront the emotions—anxiety, frustration, anger, fear, guilt, and depression—that trigger the stress response. Powerlessness often is the major culprit. Stress reduction is about gaining control of your environment, and moving from victimhood to empowerment.

[STRESS *first aid—page 213*]

RELAX

ALL WORK AND NO PLAY?... MANY OF US HAVE TO WORK HARD TO RELAX. WHATEVER IT TAKES TO WIND DOWN—A LONG HOT BATH, A HIKE IN THE WOODS, SEX, A TRASHY MOVIE—WE MUST LEARN TO FIT IT INTO OUR SCHEDULES. BECAUSE IF STRESS CAN WOUND, RELAXATION CAN HEAL. Consider this: the average American spends 9,346 hours of his life cleaning the house. The number of hours just devoted to thinking or relaxing? 3,084.

MAINTENANCE: **VISUALIZATION AND BIOFEEDBACK:** In the increasing number of stress disorder clinics popping up around the country, doctors use visualization and biofeedback techniques to teach patients how to regulate those stress responses once thought to be beyond conscious control—increased blood pressure, heart rate, respiration, muscle tension, and sweat gland activity. For example, when the body is under stress, the blood supply redistributes itself away from the extremities—hence the annoyingly cold hands and feet associated with anxiety. With biofeedback, a temperature sensor with a soft auditory tone is placed on the client's finger so she can see and hear her hand temperature. As she starts to relax—through learned techniques like deep abdominal breathing, muscle relaxation, and visualization of calming scenes—her muscles warm, and she can shut the tone off. Eventually, the client learns how to shut off stress responses without the machinery. **TRANSCENDENTAL MEDITATION:** The whole idea behind TM is the transcendence of the ordinary, noisy thoughts and emotions that crowd the brain to a place of silence and peace—a place where the brain can heal itself of the world's bruising. Indeed, studies have proven experienced TM practitioners can reduce blood pressure, reverse depression, and—while this is still a point of lively debate between Western and Eastern doctors—lower the rate of tumor growth. **EXERCISE:** Exercise may be the single most reliable form of relaxation—particularly for women, who, according to stress experts, have a higher rate of muscular problems from stress than men. So working up a sweat is fantastic for flushing out toxins from the muscles and releasing tension. But forget about the "No pain, no gain" ethos of the '80s. When it starts to hurt, quit. Even if you cannot get to the gym or out to the tennis court during the day, you can do some physical movement to help release stress. For instance, gently tensing and relaxing muscles (starting at the toes, and working upward) for 15 minutes a day will help relieve stress and improve concentration. Relax, it's your life.

W E L L N E S S

HOLISTIC MEDICINE EMBRACES A PHILOSOPHY MOST AMERICANS FIND IRRESISTIBLE: THE NOTION THAT EVERY INDIVIDUAL HAS ULTIMATE control over his or her health. In conventional, reactive medicine, the model is sickness: we feel lousy, we go to a doctor, he fixes us up, and we don't see him again until the system breaks down again. Holistic medicine, by contrast, focuses on a model of prevention, of wellness. Wellness is about caring for our bodies not solely out of fear or vanity (although both are, admittedly, good motivators), but out of a sense of pride tempered with honesty. Wellness means knowing what lengths we will go to better our health—and what lengths, for you, just aren't worth it. Maybe an extremely low-fat diet will give you a couple of extra years—but is life without clotted Devonshire cream worth living? OK, you'll give up smoking and start exercising—but maybe you're attached to a couple of Scotches after work, and those stay. In short, wellness is about choices: having the information at hand to know what's optimal, but having the common sense to know that some small pleasures supersede the demands of good health.

"To love oneself is the beginning of a lifelong romance."

OSCAR WILDE

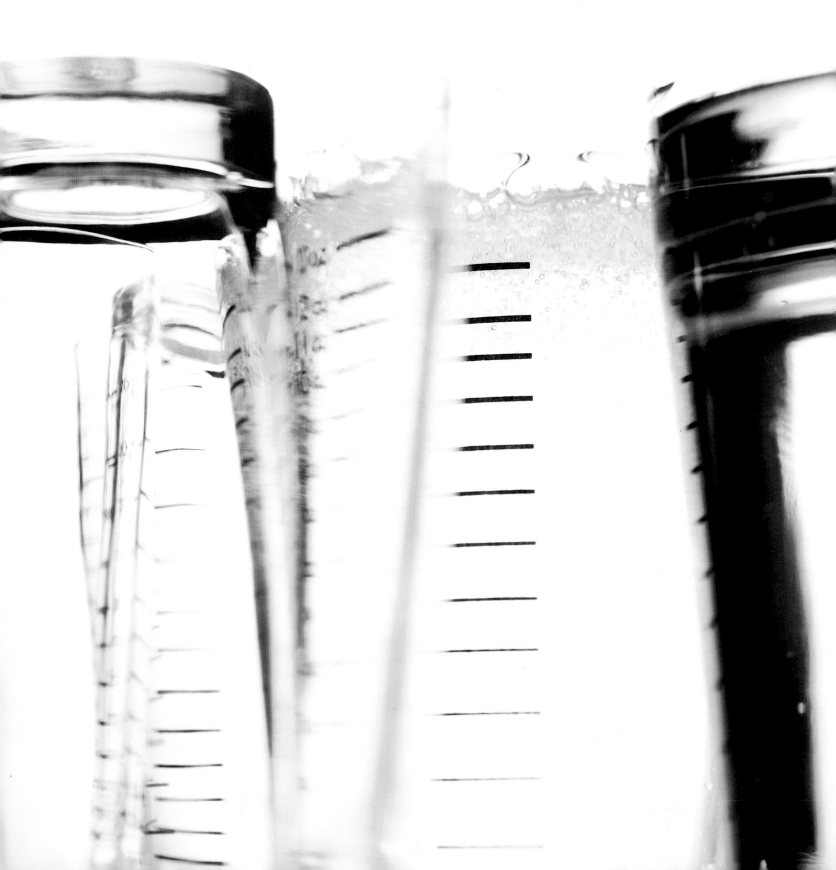

A R O M A T

"PHYSICIANS MIGHT, I BELIEVE, MAKE GREATER USE OF SCENT THAN THEY DO," WROTE THE FRENCH ESSAYIST MICHEL DE MONTAIGNE, "FOR I have often noticed that they cause changes in me and act on my spirits according to their qualities." Montaigne made this observation in 1580; it's only taken doctors and researchers 400 years to conclude he may have had a point. For centuries there's been anecdotal evidence demonstrating that smells evoke long-forgotten memories (remember Proust's madeleines?), influence our moods, and subliminally attract or repel potential mates. Only within the last decade have scientists taken these stories into the lab and attempted to prove that smells have very real physiological effects on our nervous and immune systems—effects that may eventually help us control blood pressure, reduce

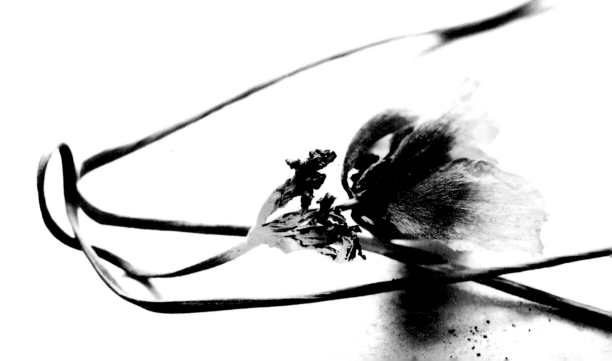

H E R A P Y

anxiety, and lift depression without drugs. Aromatherapists have made a case for the power of scents to heal. There is evidence to suggest that smells have unexplained effects on the nervous and immune systems. In 1987, a team of researchers won a "new use" patent on nutmeg oil after establishing that nutmeg, when presented alone or in a scented carrier, significantly reduced blood pressure in response to mild stress.

OPTIONS: The list of odors and their purported effects is encyclopedic: juniper, for example, helps overcome fatigue; rose cures depression and insomnia; and basil is supposed to relieve a variety of ailments, including depression, migraine, and nausea. **AROMATHERAPY AT A GLANCE:** INVIGORATING SCENTS: clove, rosemary, spruce, juniper, lemon, peppermint. STRESS RELIEVERS: vanilla, nutmeg, orange. RELAXANTS: jasmine, chamomile, marjoram, lavender, rose. APHRODISIACS: sandalwood, ylang-ylang, sage.

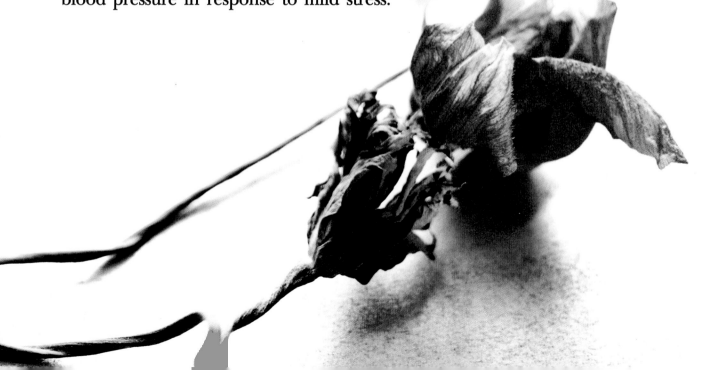

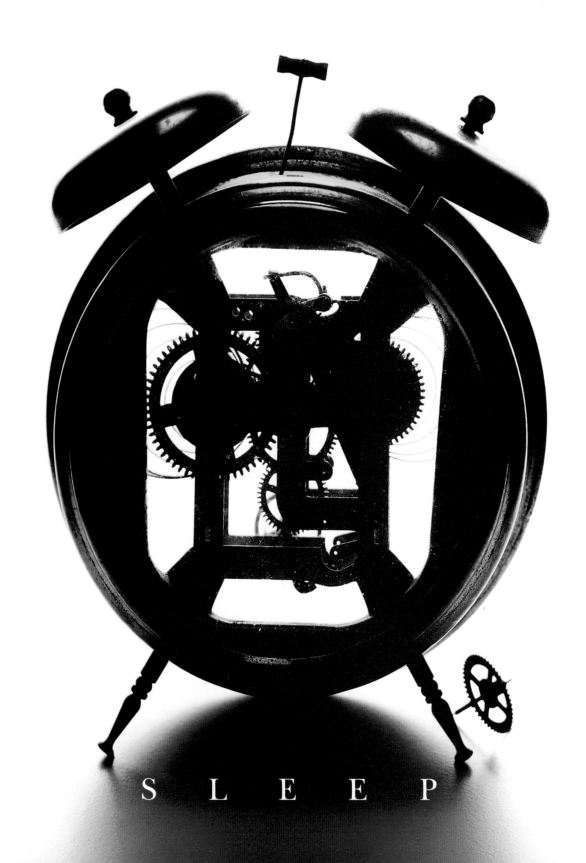

S L E E P

FROM OUR LATE-NIGHT TV JESTERS TO 24-HOUR HOME SHOPPING TO THE GROWING NUMBER OF THIRD-SHIFT WORKERS AND THE NEED TO CRAM MORE INTO EACH DAY, SLEEP IS BECOMING A DWINDLING RESOURCE. IT'S NO WONDER, THEN, THAT WHAT WEATHER IS TO ENGLAND, SLEEP IS TO AMERICA: THE PREDOMINANT topic of polite small talk over the watercooler in the morning. "How much sleep did you get last night?" "If only I could get a few extra hours"—or the annoying "I need only four hours' sleep."

MAINTENANCE: In a lifetime, the average American spends 24 years sleeping and has 1,947 nightmares. **HOW MUCH?** However much you need to function normally the next day. Some people require five hours; some require ten. As we grow older, we spend less time in stages 3 and 4, the most restful forms of sleep—which may be why older people seem to sleep less and be more tired during the day. **BETTER SLEEP:** Avoid alcohol, caffeine, and nicotine for at least four hours before bedtime. Although alcohol may initially make you sleepy, something about the metabolizing of the sugar in a drink can also wake you after a few hours. **EXERCISING:** If you're having problems getting to sleep, do not exercise at night. Working out increases energy and revs the metabolism for several hours thereafter, so people who exercise at 8:00 or 9:00 P.M. often feel like polishing the silverware around midnight. **SHEEPY:** If you can't fall asleep within 15 or 20 minutes, don't just lie there—get up, read, bake cookies. You want to associate bed with sleep—not with tossing and turning. Warm milk really does aid sleep: scientists suspect there's some protein in milk that's a relative to the protein secreted in the brain which regulates the body's sleep mechanism. Taking sleeping pills will, in the short run, make you sleep; but since they alter natural sleep patterns, over time they may actually rob you of rest and make it more difficult for you to fall asleep naturally. **SLEEP APNEA:** A common condition in overweight men over 40, where the sleeper stops breathing from 10 to 60 seconds—and breathing then resumes, usually with an enormous snort. The cause is usually folds of fat around the larynx that block the air passage. Apnea is rarely serious, and it often goes away with weight reduction.

Number of Americans who sleep in pajamas
32,932,623 (men)
17,744,653 (women)

Number who sleep in underwear
29,372,339 (men)
3,735,716 (women)

Number who sleep in the nude
16,911,347 (men)
5,603,575 (women)

Number of women who sleep in nighties/nightgowns
58,837,534

Number of Americans who say they dream while sleeping
124 million

Number who say they dream in color
50 million
in black and white
29 million

[🛏 SLEEP *first aid—page 213*]

BETTY FRIEDAN

What Betty Friedan's *The Feminine Mystique* did for women, her recent *The Fountain of Age* does for aging. Citing often surprising statistics, she debunks the "old" stereotypes of sexless, feeble-minded cranks, most of whom end up in nursing homes. Simultaneously, through interviews with myriad older men and women, she

"I began to recognize some people who had crossed the
hood, some strength or
going and growing. It sur
I dreaded doing those inter
to wallow personally in the
really want to look at or
old people. Even

stresses the real benefits of growing older: the chance to do what
Friedan calls "human work," work
you've always wanted to do but
never had time for: to form strong
bonds with family and friends; to
discover real sexual intimacy. But,

Friedan stresses, none of this is
possible without a change in attitude toward growing old: "Aging
is an adventure," says Friedan. An
adventure only if our individual
and societal perceptions recognize
it as an estimable stage of one's life.

new dimension of person-
quality of being in
chasm of age—and kept on
prised me. To be honest,
views at first. I had no wish
dreariness of age..I didn't
listen to those finished
'vital' ones.

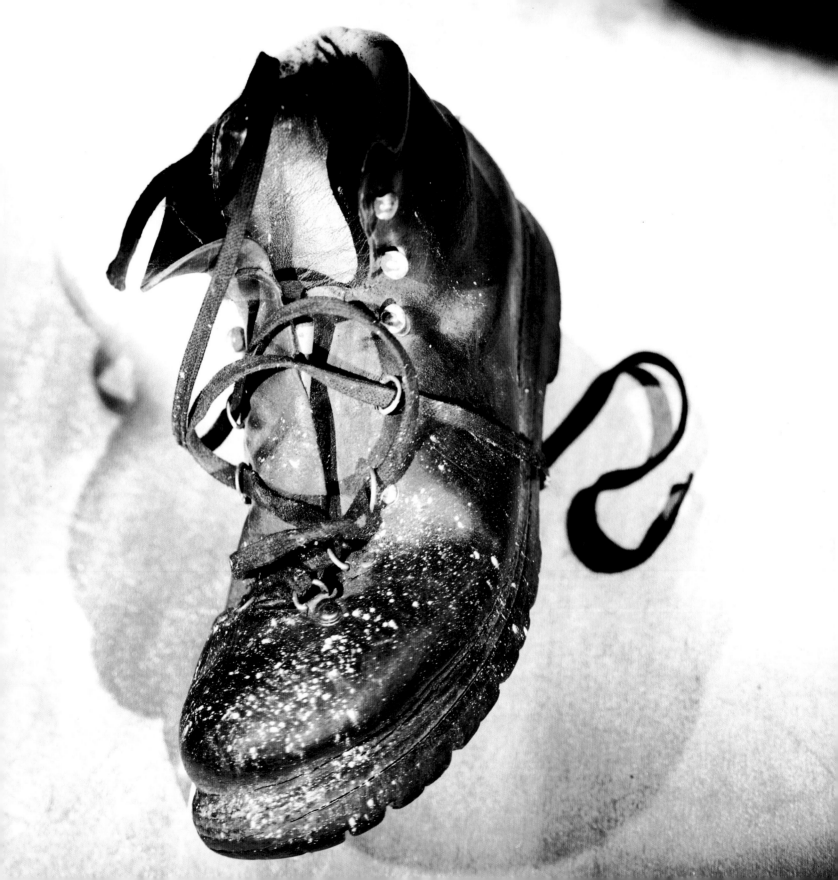

FITNESS

HIGH-IMPACT EXERCISERS WHO DO RUNNING, SWIMMING, AND AEROBICS HAVE BUTTED HEADS WITH LOW-IMPACT EXERCISERS WHO PREFER yoga, ballet positions, orthopedic exercises, and muscle conditioning over a key question: do you need pain to gain? The answer, it appears, is no, as exercise researchers have discovered getting fit isn't quite the Sisyphean task it was reckoned to be in the '80s. The key to fitness is consistency, not intensity. Merely burning 2,000 extra calories a week—which can be accomplished by walking an hour a day—helps protect against cardiovascular disease. And the exercise does not have to take place during one time period: three 10-minute runs a day produce nearly the same health benefits as one 30-minute run. But remember, you still have to do it.

MAINTENANCE: Fitness researchers recommend a combination of aerobic with anaerobic activity. Aerobic means the body utilizes lots of oxygen, pumping up the heart rate and burning fat; anaerobic exercise—weight training, for example—is ideal for building muscle and overall body strength, and an increase in muscle density boosts your body's metabolic rate. One type of exercise is not a substitute for the other; both are necessary.

"You have to stay in shape. My grandmother, she started walking five miles a day when she was 60. She's 97 today and we don't know where the hell she is."

ELLEN DeGENERES

E A T I N G

AMERICANS PROBABLY RECEIVE MORE INFORMATION ABOUT FOOD AND EATING THAN ANY SINGLE SUBJECT. IF ONLY WE PAID AS MUCH ATTENTION TO WHAT WE FED OUR MINDS AS WHAT WE FED OUR BODIES. WE ARE NOW BEING TOLD, "DON'T WORRY ABOUT CUTTING CALORIES, BUT CUT DOWN FAT BY 40 percent. If we could cut down by even to 20 or 25 percent, we'd be significantly reducing our chances of contracting a wide variety of diseases linked, directly or indirectly, to high fat intake— including arteriosclerosis, high blood pressure, heart disease, diabetes, and breast cancer.

MAINTENANCE: Eating well appears simple—three cups of pesticide-free vegetables; two fruits; six or seven fiber servings (two with each meal—pasta, whole wheat bread, corn, potatoes); three to four ounces of protein with each meal—preferably nonfat cheese, lean veal, nonfat yogurt, chicken breasts, tofu. Stay away from processed foods. Yet food is a major temptation and source of frustration in our society. **TIMING:** When we eat is almost as important as what we eat. Go-go Americans prefer a quick bite for breakfast and lunch, and save the groaning board for dinner at 7:00 or 8:00 P.M.—precisely the time when the food has nowhere to go, except your hips and belly. We need most of our energy, and hence our food intake, at the beginning of the day; ideally, breakfast should be the largest meal, and dinner more of a snack. **SET WEIGHT POINT?** Scientists are hotly debating the wisdom of gaining a bit of weight as we get older. Although obesity is associated with long lists of health risks, so is being underweight (pneumonia, influenza, and osteoporosis disproportionately hit the skinny). One school of thought says that it's not only safe, but preferable, to gain up to a full pound a year after forty. Many of us want to enroll in this school. Another school cites a study that shows that semistarved rats live 50 percent longer than well-fed rats—and this study, so the argument goes, also pertains to humans. Yes, but you don't see volunteers lining up to test this hypothesis, do you?

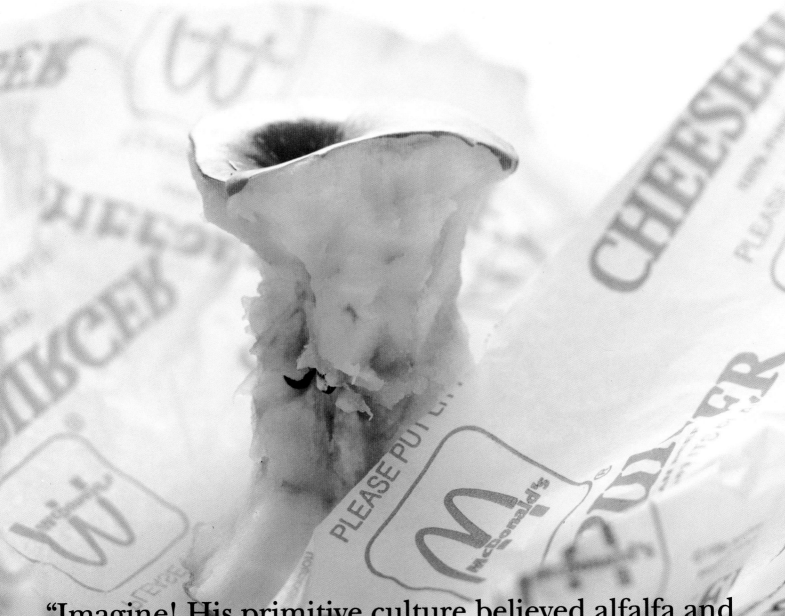

"Imagine! His primitive culture believed alfalfa and wheat germ were good for you, rather than steak and chocolate, as we know now."

SCIENTISTS MARVELING AT WOODY ALLEN'S NAIVETÉ IN THE 1973 MOVIE *SLEEPER*

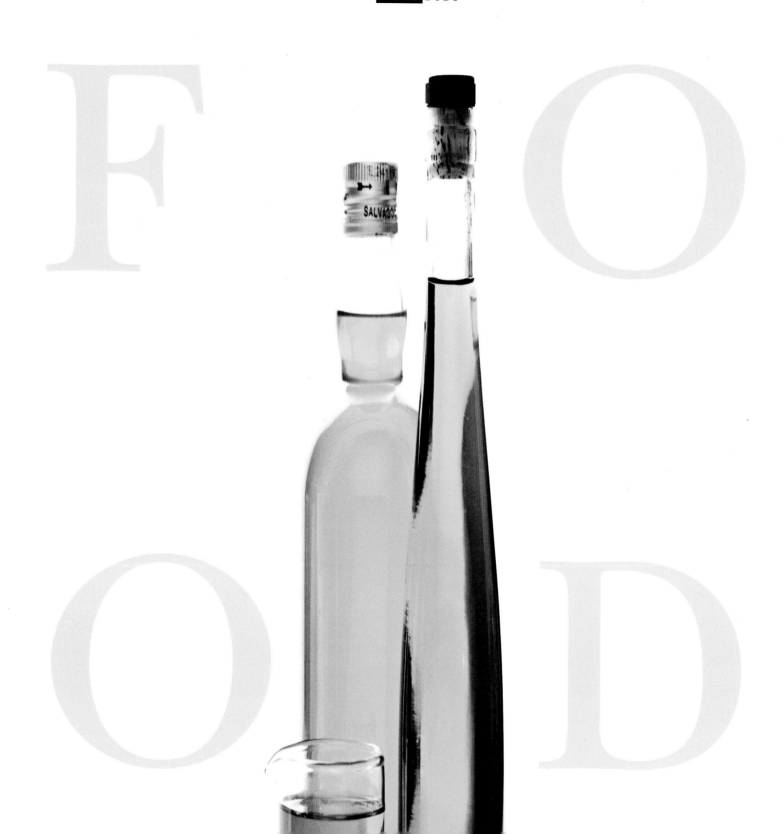

FOOD

DIET CAN'T SOLVE ALL OUR HEALTH PROBLEMS, BUT EVERY DAY WE'RE LEARNING NEW THINGS ABOUT WHAT IT CAN DO. RESEARCHERS ARE discovering not only which foods not to eat but also the foods that promote longevity. The National Cancer Institute is funding studies of cancer-inhibiting foods such as garlic (and its relatives, onion and leek), licorice root, citrus fruits, umbelliferous vegetables (the celery/parsley family), and flaxseed. The federal government is researching "nutraceuticals," the name coined for food fortified with disease-fighting substances. The U.S. Food and Drug Administration allows few food products to make medicinal claims, but in other countries, foods are allowed to tout their healing properties. Germany has snack foods containing echinacea, an herb reputed to boost the immune system. And in France, a beer that contains an herbal mixture reputed to boost the libido is sold.

Yet for every astonishing new discovery there's another report proving that yesterday's gospel truth is today's Big Lie. High cholesterol? Terrible, right? However, studies in both monkeys and humans reveal that low cholesterol levels lead to increased aggression. Humans with low cholesterol may be less likely to die of heart disease, but more likely to die of trauma-related injuries. Calcium? Osteoporosis, brought on by lack of calcium in the diet, is still a scourge of maturing women. Now some foods, like brands of orange juice, are regularly fortified with calcium. The problem here is that too much calcium in the diet can lead to kidney stones. And what about oat bran? Miracle food or merely nature's Drāno? It's undeniably an excellent source of roughage, but the oat bran fad began to fade when further studies cast doubt on its cholesterol-lowering abilities and manufacturers discovered no one liked the taste of the stuff anyway.

[FOOD *first aid—page 213*]

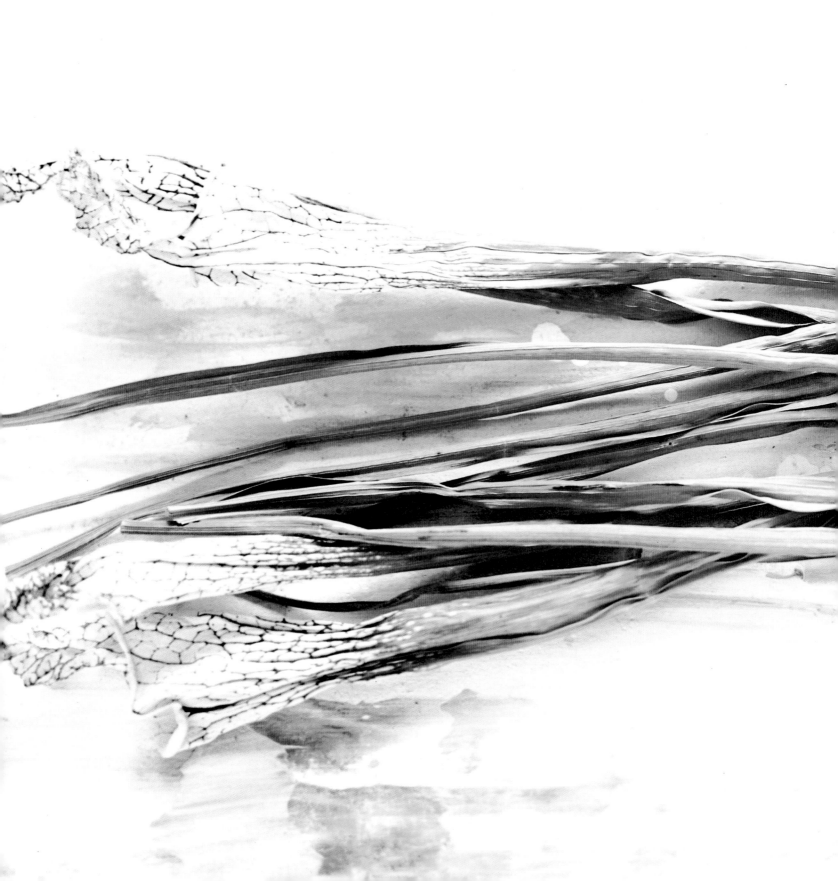

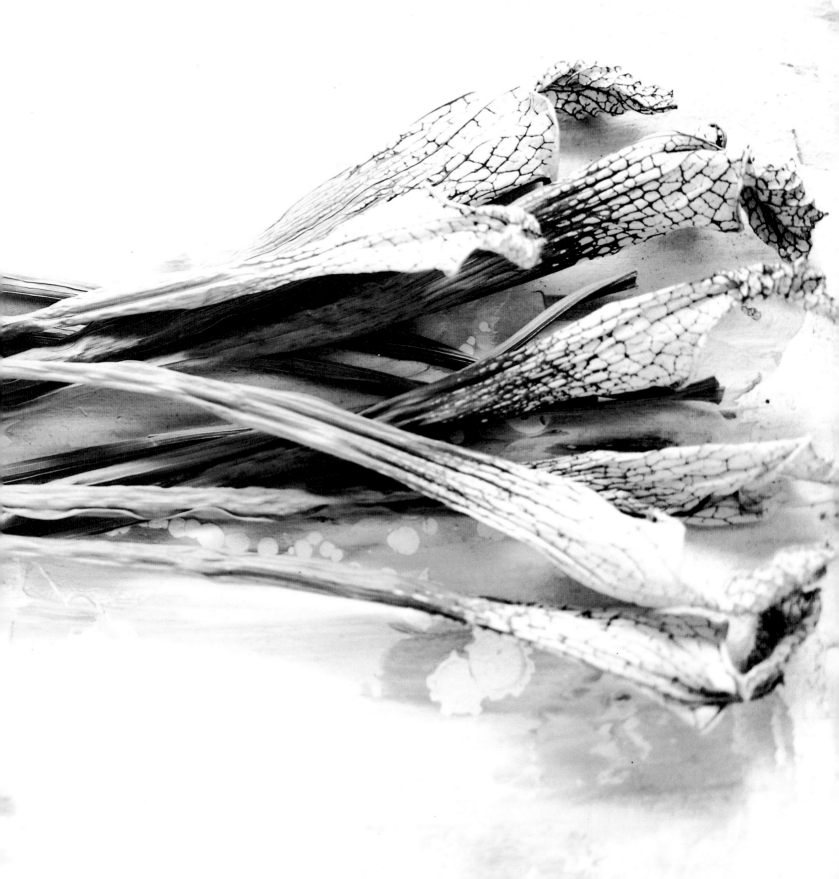

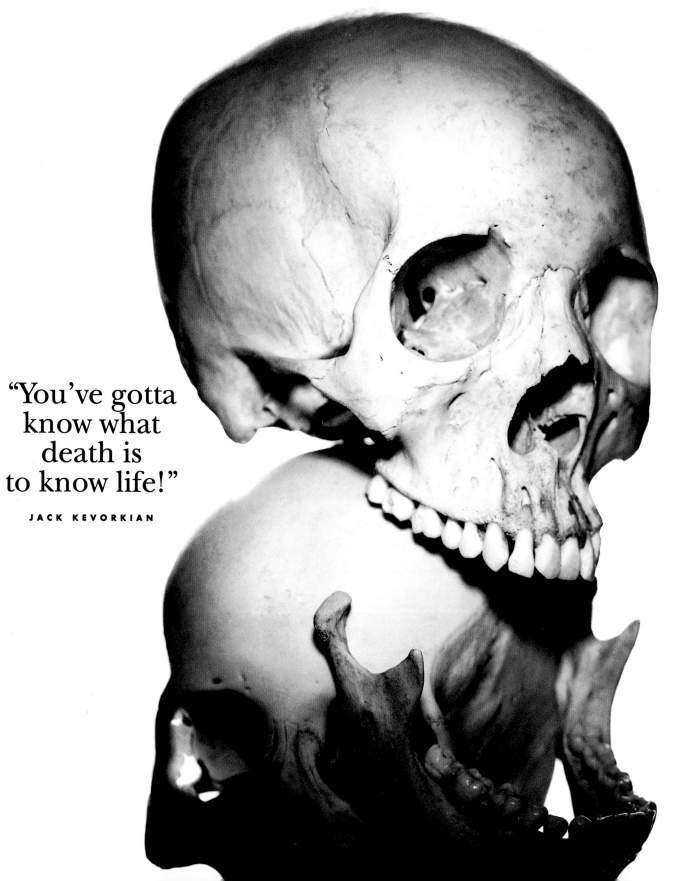

"You've gotta
know what
death is
to know life!"

JACK KEVORKIAN

L I F E

MOST OF US, NO MATTER HOW OLD WE ARE, HAVE NEVER SEEN A PERSON DIE. WE HAVE PROBABLY ALL WITNESSED LIFE'S OTHER MILE-STONES—BIRTH (AT LEAST, WE'VE SEEN IT ON TELEVISION), MARRIAGE, TAXES. BUT EVEN THOSE OF US WHO ASPIRE TO RICH EMOTIONAL LIVES SHIELD OURSELVES utterly from death. As the anthropologist Margaret Mead once noted: "When a person is born we rejoice, and when they're married we jubilate, but when they die we try to pretend nothing has happened." It follows that a country so youth-obsessed wants to keep itself death-ignorant and yearn for the Faustian legend of youth without measure.

DEATH—WHAT IT IS. Consider the oddity of this: our definition of death is changing. Every thanatologist agrees death means the end of something—but what? For centuries, death was the end of breathing and heartbeat. But in the 1950s, technology was developed that could breathe for us. In the '60s, the popular definition, proposed by Harvard Medical School, became "brain death"—complete unawareness of external stimuli, no spontaneous breathing, and a flat brain wave. But even this definition is subject to interpretation. This new definition of death has meant that life itself is also being redefined. The largest group ever to be born at one time in history will also become the largest group coming to a confrontation with death. This along with the tragedy of younger deaths owing to AIDS means that it has become more difficult to live without being constantly reminded of the inevitable. An entire industry has sprung up around our national desire to euphemize The End. We have made death, American style, into our final act of vanity, for what is vanity, after all, if not the desire to make a good impression?

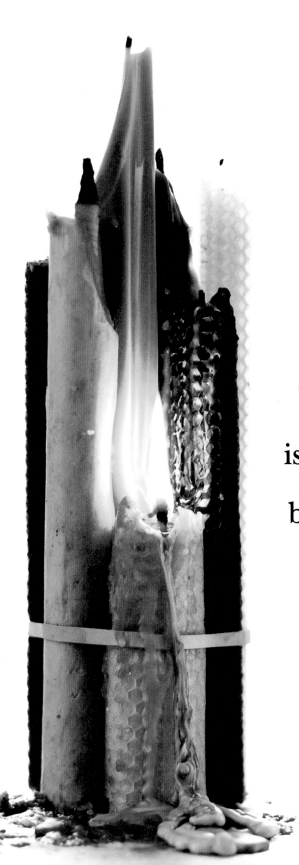

"I postpone
death by living,
by suffering,
by error, by
risking, by giving,
by losing."

ANAÏS NIN

"Life is trouble;
only death
is not. To be alive
is to undo your
belt and look for
trouble."

NIKOS KAZANTZAKIS

first aid.

As time goes by, our bodies will be exposed to a gamut of elements that will bring us both joy and grief. Our bodies are destined to change. No amount of grooming or fine-tuning will prevent the aging process. But we can learn to take better care of ourselves, to look at our bodies with more kindness, and to improve upon our current condition.

"Anatomy is destiny." SIGMUND FREUD

Heart

PULSE METERS. Most people can find their pulse by lightly resting the tips of the first two fingers on the radial artery at the wrist or the carotid artery at the neck, then counting the pulsations for ten seconds and multiplying by six to get the number of beats per minute. If you press too hard on the pulse, the heart will automatically slow down, giving you an inaccurate reading. Knowing your heart rate during exercise helps you stay in the aerobic target zone, where heart and lungs must work hard to meet the increased demand for oxygen. If you are a die-hard exerciser and have a hard time finding your pulse fifteen seconds after you exercise, pulse meters are devices that will give you exact pulse figures, target time zones for reaching prime aerobic peaks, and records of the heart pattern during recovery time. Are they worth it? If you feel your heart pumping hard for more than twenty minutes, you can be convinced that you have gained aerobic benefits, despite what your pulse may be telling you. Pulse meters were originally intended for use by patients with heart problems who need to keep track of their pulse for medical purposes.

EXERCISE. Aerobic activity is not enough. Strength training is also necessary for keeping the heart healthy. See the exercise chapter for more information.

FAILURE. A heart attack or cardiac arrest occurs when the blood vessels (arteries) which supply oxygen to the heart muscle become obstructed or blocked. This happens over a period of time, and many victims of heart attacks often ignore the warning signs that arise before their hearts stop beating. The most common signals are a pressure or sense of fullness in your chest, often described as a tightness, burning, aching, or crushing pain, abnormal feelings of breathlessness, weakness, or tiredness, a stabbing pain that radiates down your limbs, across your shoulders, and up your neck and jaw (watch out especially for pain in your left arm), sweating, or nausea. Any of these signs should warrant a doctor's visit. Delaying medical treatment when these signs manifest themselves decreases your chances of surviving a heart attack. Fact: Per capita, the French, known for their high-fat diets, drink nine times as much wine as Americans do, but their rate of death from heart disease is significantly lower.

Apparently, alcohol is like Drāno for the blood vessels. It keeps platelets—the small cells in the blood that form a clot to stop the bleeding from a wound—from narrowing veins and arteries dangerously.

CPR. HOW TO GIVE CPR IF YOU ARE ALONE WITH A HEART ATTACK VICTIM. This is scary stuff, but screaming and panicking is not going to help. Try to remain calm and focused. Remember, you are the victim's life-cord until other help arrives. The main purpose of CPR is to keep the lungs supplied with oxygen, and to keep the blood circulating to the heart, brain, and other vital body parts. Bear in mind that after four minutes, the brain will start deteriorating from lack of oxygen; every second counts—there is no time for hysteria.

HOW TO DO IT:

1. Gently shake the victim and ask, "Are you OK?" to see if the victim is alert. If there is no response, immediately check his pulse at the neck for five to ten seconds (to find someone's pulse at the neck, take your index and middle finger and place it on the neck right above the Adam's apple). At the same time, look, listen, and feel for breathing—

look at the patient's chest to see if he's breathing, put your ear to his nose and mouth to listen, and feel for breath. If you find a pulse, but the patient is not breathing, clear his air passage by tilting the head up so the chin is higher than the heart. Check again to see if breathing has resumed. If you don't feel any breath coming out, pinch the nose, keep the chin raised, and place your mouth over the patient's mouth, making sure you make a tight seal so none of the oxygen you give escapes. Then give two quick deep breaths followed by one breath every five seconds at the rate of one to one and one half seconds per breath. Try to get help immediately.

2. If the patient shows no sign of a pulse and is not breathing, then his heart has stopped beating, and you must begin CPR. Kneel at the side of the patient's body so your head is looking across the victim's chest. With your right hand place your index and middle fingers at the bottom of his sternum (you can find the sternum by running your hand down the rib cage until you feel the last bone—this is the sternum). Then place the heel of your left hand right above your two fingers. Your right hand should now go directly over the left, and your fingers should be interlocked. Keeping your elbows straight and locked, use the force of your body to push the heel of your hand straight down and up. Do not bend your elbows. The compressions should be in the middle of the chest. If you bend your elbows to give force to your compressions, the movement will not be effective. Each compression should go about one and one half to two inches into the chest. Pressing too hard could break the ribs, so be forceful but don't overdo it. You should compress 15 times in a row, counting "one–one thousand, two–one thousand," as you compress. After the 15 pushes, you must give two breaths to the mouth, remembering to tilt the head back to open the passageway, and to pinch the nostrils to keep oxygen from escaping. Repeat this pattern until help

arrives, or the victim regains his pulse or breathing. Giving CPR is easier if two people are involved. If another person can assist you, have him either do the compressing or the breathing. If two people are administering CPR the ratio would be 5 chest compressions for every breath.

Digestive

GAS. Digested carbohydrates migrate from the stomach, where carbohydrates are rarely digested and absorbed, to the lower intestine, where they encounter families of bacteria that continue the digestive process. These bacteria feed on undigested carbohydrates, releasing gas in the process. When you're going to, say, the boss's house for dinner, avoid eating broccoli, Brussels sprouts, cabbage, or milk products beforehand. Eat and drink slowly, chewing your food; don't eat a lot of products with chemical sweeteners like sorbitol—they cause gas and are difficult to digest.

ULCERS. Experiencing discomfort after eating, or a general gassy or burning feeling in the stomach area, does not mean you have an ulcer. What you are probably experiencing is indigestion, a very common condition that will go away by itself. Taking an over-the-counter medication will help to relieve discomfort. When should you worry? If your tummy is gassy or burns daily, and the pain remains consistent whether you eat or not, this may be a good time to consult with a doctor. Ulcers, often thought to be stress-related, are generally not. They are tiny open wounds on the stomach lining which, when exposed to the acids in the stomach, can cause a great deal of pain. There is speculation that ulcers are exacerbated by a kind of bacteria. Medication can be prescribed for treatment. Several ways to minimize risk of ulcers: **1.** Don't smoke—smokers are twice as likely to have peptic ulcers. **2.** Don't overuse aspirin. People who take four or more aspirin a day for three or more months increase their chance of getting an ulcer.

CHOKING. If you don't already know, the universal sign for choking is the clasping of the hands around the neck. It sounds obvious, but when treating a choking victim, it is important to differentiate someone who is choking and cannot breathe from someone who has something caught in his throat and is coughing to remove it. If the person has partial airway blockage and is coughing, his air exchange is good enough for him to remove the object by himself. While this may be difficult to watch, it is best to leave him alone and encourage continued coughing. Do not perform the Heimlich maneuver. However, if the person is clasping his hands around his throat, has a weak, ineffective cough, and is making a high-pitched noise while trying to breathe, he has either total blockage of the airway or partial blockage with poor air exchange. Performing the Heimlich maneuver in this case is necessary. Here's how you do it:

1. Ask the person if he's choking to make sure he's not just laughing or playing a joke.

2. If he nods yes, stand behind the victim and wrap your arms around his waist.

3. Make a fist with one hand, then place the thumb side of the fist on the abdomen so the thumb is touching right above the navel and below the tip of the breastbone.

4. Grasp the fist with your other hand, keeping your elbows away from the person as you press your fist into the person's abdomen with a quick upward thrust. Make sure the fist is in the midline of the abdomen when you press. Don't direct the thrusts to the right or left.

5. Continue to repeat thrusts until the obstruction is cleared and the person resumes breathing. If you hear the victim coughing after thrusts have been made, leave him alone, and allow him to remove the obstruction himself.

6. If the person becomes unconscious, then quickly perform rescue breathing (see under CPR, in the Heart section of this book).

FOR YOUNG CHILDREN:

7. Turn the child over on his stomach on your lap so his head is facing downwards. Strike him with the heel of your hand in an upward motion between the shoulder blades.

Bones

ENEMIES OF CALCIUM. Caffeine, salt, certain medications (like antacids and some diuretics), and lack of exercise all contribute to calcium loss.

THE MAGNESIUM FACTOR. It's unclear exactly how the two work together, but magnesium helps us absorb calcium into our bones, increasing our bone density. Magnesium-rich foods include grains, bananas, spinach, and other dark green vegetables. (But beware of magnesium supplements: they can act like laxatives.)

Brain

AVOIDING MIGRAINES. Certain foods seem to trigger them: aged cheese, freshly baked bread, red wine, chocolate, nuts, MSG, and bacon. At least one recent study proved that taking an aspirin a day can reduce migraine frequency.

SMART DRUGS. Pushing aside all their bad press, what are "smart drugs" anyway, and do they work? It depends who you ask. Often associated with the rave culture and technophiles, smart drugs are said to improve memory, concentration, alertness, problem-solving ability, and—here's the biggie—delay the cognitive effects of aging. These drugs sometimes appear in liquid form under names such as Fast Blast and Energy Elixir, and are served in health food bars and popular clubs around the country. The medical establishment has been using these nootropics (the medical term for cognitive-enhancer drugs) on patients suffering from Alzheimer's disease, strokes, and senile dementia abroad, but their use hasn't really caught on in this country. Although many of these drugs originated in the U.S.—such as hydergine, which physicians tried with apparent lack of success on patients suffering from Alzheimer's disease—the medical establishment in this country is still reluctant to use them. But many people are using these smart drugs to improve their already well-functioning brain—to become smarter. Using drugs to enhance brain capacity strikes a skeptical chord among many doctors. However, those who have used them claim they become more alert and aware after using them. Some advocates of smart drugs report having more energy, which differs from feeling smarter. This would make sense when you consider that caffeine is often a prime ingredient in smart drinks. The idea of taking a drug to make you smarter and to cancel the effects of debilitating diseases is a remarkably seductive one, and one that will probably not fade away without a good fight.

CONCUSSIONS. Concussions are bruises of the brain, and occur when there is a forceful blow or impact to the head. Usually, patients will be nauseated, feel dizzy, and sometimes lose consciousness. Mild concussions require medical attention. People will often misdiagnose themselves when they have suffered a significant blow to the head, and go about their daily routine. It is crucial to be examined by a doctor because if there is swelling of the brain, it could be life-threatening. If you have suffered a head injury, no matter how minor, see a doctor immediately to get a full examination.

Facial Skin

ACNE. Unfortunately, acne does not stop after puberty. When breakouts are frequent, consult a dermatologist. Don't leave your face in the hands of the blemish banishers. Most cases of acne are easily treatable by prescriptive drugs; Accutane, Retin-A, and AHA all have high success rates. For occasional blemishes, stick to your cleansing routine, and eventually they should clear up. Sometimes, relieving the pressure and buildup of a pimple by gently squeezing it can help it go away faster. Your mother always told you to just leave it alone, but squeezing the pimple can actually speed up recovery time. Don't oversqueeze. If the pimple doesn't seem like it will open, leave it alone. Oversqueezing can scar the face, so use a light touch.

"Is that a beard, or are you eating a muskrat?"

DR. GONZO

SUNBURN. Misery is the best deterrent from getting sunburned twice. Sunscreen is a must when you're in the sun. Here's how to quell a sunburn: Start with any cooling lotion, cool compresses, or a cool bath. Use a moisturizing lotion to minimize burning and skin tightness. Don't open any blisters that might appear. As they break naturally, apply an over-the-counter antiseptic like Neosporin or Polysporin, and then cover the exposed areas so they don't get dirty. While researchers aren't convinced of aloe vera's effectiveness, this product seems to soothe inflammation, inhibit swelling, and allow blood to reach the injured tissue. When looking for cooling lotions, choose one that contains 70 percent aloe vera. Sunburn, depending on the degree, usually takes two to five days to clear.

PH BALANCE. **WHAT IS PH BALANCE?** It is the skin's natural defense system that fights off bacteria and holds the right amount of moisture to keep the skin healthy. The chemical makeup of the skin ranges between acidity and alkalinity. Ideally, the skin's pH is around 5.5, the midway point between these two chemical levels. Healthy skin does not need to be pH-balanced. It naturally leans to the acidic side of the scale because it produces a protective layer of bacteria (called the acid mantle) which wards off unfriendly bacteria and seals in moisture. More important are the skin products you use which could disturb your natural pH. Stick to a minimal number of products, and stop using any product that irritates your skin. Any tingling sensation that arises after skin cleansing means your skin is begging you, "Please stop using that product—it hurts." If the pH balance is disturbed by skin-care products, the acid mantle will break down, allowing bacteria to penetrate the skin's surface, causing infection. But once disturbed, the skin has an amazing capacity to return to normal pH levels in just eight hours. Acned skin and extra-dry skin might take longer to recover from an off-kilter pH. Alkali, a common ingredient in cleansers, can provoke these skin conditions, so it is best to avoid products containing it. What about all those products promising a perfect pH? If they work, fine. Do you need them? Probably not. Are we going to tell you what to do? Definitely not. Note: The eye moisturizers, gels, or makeup removers that you use around your eyes may cause eye irritation if their pH is different from the pH of your tears, so take precautions.

FEMALE FACIAL SKIN. Women often purchase the wrong products for their skin type; too much of a good thing can cause dry skin, acne, or oily skin. Heavy moisturizers, for example, can clog pores, causing breakouts. Facial masks can rob the skin of its own natural moisture, leaving it dry. Harsh blemish medication can irritate your pimples even more. The fewer products you use in your skin-care routine, the better off your skin will feel and look.

FEMALE DRY SKIN. Avoid using washcloths, tissues, hot water, dry saunas, or skin-care products containing anything irritating or drying, like soap (use a water-soluble cleanser instead). Dry skin will not go away by using greasy or thick products; they will only make the skin look dull, and cause breakouts. It is a myth that people with dry skin wrinkle faster than those with normal to oily skin. Don't be seduced by the cosmetic hype that tells you otherwise; it will leave your wallet empty and your shelves filled with moisturizers in pretty bottles that you

don't need. People with dry skin need to moisturize during the day and before going to sleep. If possible, purchase a moisturizer with sunscreen for the day, and another one for the evening. Ingredients to ignore when choosing skin-care products for dry skin include: amniotic fluid, animal tissue extract, algae extract, and indeed all products containing extracts of any kind. Ingredients to look for: allantoin, alpha hydroxy acids, amino acids, avocado oil, collagen, egg oil, coconut oil.

"A woman has the age she deserves."

COCO CHANEL

FEMALE OILY SKIN. Avoid using products that claim they will dry out blemishes or absorb oil. For anyone over 18, these products will only irritate your skin. To combat oily skin, follow a simple and gentle skin-care routine, as described in the maintenance section. Many cosmetic products intended for oily skin contain alcohol, which is irritating; products labeled as "non-greasy" or "hypo-allergenic" should be avoided. Oily skin moisturizes itself, and does not require any more moisture. Ingredients to avoid: salicyclic acid, benzoyl peroxide, sulfur, boric acid, and clove oil. Ingredients to look for include: allantoin, alpha hydroxy acids, bentonite, and glycerin.

MALE FACIAL SKIN. Taking care of male skin means going beyond shaving practices and techniques. Men are now offered full skin-care lines—for dry or oily skin—especially geared to the needs of male skin.

MALE DRY SKIN. Say good-bye to washing your face in the shower with the same soap you use on your body. Soap may contribute to your problem; use a water-soluble cleanser instead. If you don't want to give up your old habit, at least opt for a super-fatted soap that is gentler on the skin. Even if you never dreamed of using it or don't think you need it, a moisturizer is a must after you shave if your skin is dry. There are plenty of moisturizers and aftershave lotions on the market for men that are scent-free and inexpensive, so save your skin and use them. You don't need to spend a lot of money on a moisturizer to get good results. Experiment with some cheap products, and if they work you can use them on any part of your body that feels dry. The best way to apply a moisturizing product is to put it on damp, not wet, skin. Avoid mineral oil in your moisturizing products because it will absorb your natural oils and increase dryness. When choosing a shaving cream, the basic rule is to use a cream or lotion with an oil base.

MALE OILY SKIN. Face brushes work wonders on oily skin. They are small, inexpensive products with small bristles that are terrific for cleansing the skin and lessening the frequency of breakouts. Choose a standard shaving-cream product that is rich in silicone. You do not need to apply a moisturizer, since your skin already produces enough of its own oils. However, it's a good idea to apply a small amount of moisturizer if areas of your face are dry—the forehead and the area around the eyes are common trouble spots.

TIPS:

1. If you've had a rough night, running an ice cube over your cheeks and around the eyes will tighten the skin and give it a glow. But don't do this often since it can damage the capillaries.

2. To perk up lifeless skin, use a scrub lotion to make skin look fresher. Don't use it more than twice a week, or when you have a tan.

3. Try to avoid touching your face throughout the day. Many times when we experience stress or anxiety we will rub our hands on our face, making it more dirty and oily.

4. Get into the habit of washing your face when you come home from work. This will eliminate the possibility of falling asleep on the couch in front of the television before you give your face a proper cleaning.

Makeup

SHOPPING FOR MAKEUP. Shopping for makeup can be almost as agonizing as buying a bathing suit. When shopping for cosmetics, never buy products you don't need, don't like, or can't afford. Bring a friend along to restrain you if you're easily seduced by salespeople behind cosmetic counters. If all else fails, most cosmetic companies will accept returns or exchanges. If the salesperson gives you a hard time, you should write to the cosmetic company and it likely will refund your purchase.

TO HELP AVOID THIS INCONVENIENCE:

1. Beware of the store's interior lighting. Cosmetic mirrors at the counter are designed to flatter. Walk outside before purchasing any makeup product to check the color in daylight.
2. Also ask to see if you can get a sample product that you can try at home.
3. Keep in mind that the salesperson is not a voice of authority or wisdom. You are your own expert. Their job is to sell their products to you, so if they recommend a lipstick color that you know makes your skin look green, just say no. Go with your gut instincts when it comes to choosing colors you like to wear. You know

"Beauty will not season soup."

POLISH PROVERB

what flatters you the most. Stick with this internal radar and most of your cosmetic purchases will be successful.

4. When shopping for foundation, don't wear your own foundation to the store.
5. More than two shades of any color of lipstick or blush is a waste of money. You don't need five shades of red lipstick. Find two that you love and stick with them.
6. A good cosmetic product does not have to be expensive. Paying more money for a product does not guarantee its value. Some expensive products might be better than others, but generally the formulas used are the same. If you swear by a certain line and the color range it offers, by all means continue using those products. Women often spend more money on lipstick and mascara in department stores than they need to. Drugstore cosmetics can work just as well. The drawback to shopping at a drugstore is that you have to wait to go home to see how the product will look. Lipsticks, eye shadows, and foundation are the most difficult products to buy at drugstores simply because you can't try them on; often you can't even see the true color of the product. If you already know what colors look best on your lips, drugstores are the best place to shop. Drugstore eye shadows tend to be too shiny, and the color selection is often limited. Foundation is nearly impossible to buy at the drugstore. Some cosmetic lines offer foundation testers, but if you can't try it on or see how it looks in daylight, don't buy it. The best bets for drugstore purchases are mascaras, eyeliners, and lip liners. Drugstore mascaras can be just as good as the brands at the department stores. The quality of lip liners and eyeliners is standard; they should not cost you more than five dollars.

CHOOSING COLORS. Forget spring colors or fall colors or colors to wear at night, or for work, or to go with a certain blouse. What is most flattering to your face, your skin complexion, and your facial features should always determine how you choose your makeup colors. Every season, the word is out on what colors are in for the cheeks, lips, and eyes. For the most part, ignore all this information. Most

models will look good no matter what makeup they are wearing. There is a difference between knowing what is fashionable and being a slave to fashion. You have the power to decide what colors work best for you—not the cosmetic industry. In the end, how one chooses to paint one's face is a matter of choice. We do not hold the answer; we only offer our advice. Here are some suggestions:

1. Daytime makeup should be soft, and on the natural side.
2. Evening makeup should be more dramatic. The reasons are pretty straightforward: daytime light is stronger than evening's dimmer light, and thus makeup should be worn accordingly.
3. Only one feature should be accentuated at a time. If you want to accentuate the lips, go easy on the eye shadow. Dramatic eyes call for muted lips, and so forth.
4. Colors to avoid: just say no to fluorescent orange lipstick, heavy matte eye shadow (unless you want to look sleep-deprived), to electric blue or green eyeliner worn alone, to white lip gloss, to blue or shiny metallic eye shadows. Note: Older women, especially, should take precautions when choosing makeup colors. Shiny eye shadows will accentuate any fine lines around the eyes, and make lids look wrinkled. Most makeup artists agree that older women should not use more makeup to cover wrinkles or aging signs. It is a natural tendency for women to want to cover the changes in their face, but foundation and concealer, if applied too heavily, will give a mummified effect.

FOUNDATION. The color of foundation is supposed to match the skin exactly. There should be no color difference between the neck and the foundation. Experts warn against foundations that are too pink, green, orange, peach, rose, ashy, or yellow. No matter what your skin color, foundation should be a neutral shade of ivory, to tan, to dark brown, to ebony. Foundation should be invisible but provide coverage. The texture should be soft and smooth, and should not look cakey, unnatural, or thick. Finding the perfect foundation takes time, so have patience. Certain cosmetic lines can mix a personalized foundation color for you. Some strategies to check color. Stripe a foundation color on the side of your face, then wait a minute for it to dry to see if it blends with your skin color. If the color is right, you should not see a stain on the face. Check the shade under different lights, especially fluorescent light, because makeup may look gray under the blue undertones of fluorescent light.

CONCEALER. When trying to hide pimples, use concealers with a green/blue hue so they will cancel out the red look of the skin underneath. When trying to cover circles under the eyes, your best bet is to find a product that is close to your skin tone, or even slightly yellow. Overcorrecting with a color that is too pale will draw attention to the problem and make you look sickly. Note: Remember that concealer and foundation must blend. Any concealer tone that is nonneutral will change the shade of foundation around the eyes. Choose a concealer one or two shades lighter than the foundation to avoid problems. Ignore products called "color correctors." That's marketing psychobabble, not an actual cosmetic tool. Just stick with a foundation and concealer in the proper color.

FORMULAS. Choosing a foundation formula is a personal decision. There is no right or wrong formula. You should keep your skin type in mind when deciding.
1. Mousses and foams require little blending and feel weightless, but don't give much coverage.
2. Stick foundations give lots of coverage but require primers before application. They are also tricky to put on smoothly.
3. Tinted moisturizers combine skin care, sun protection, and foundation, yet the color range is very limited.
4. Cream formulas are great for dry skin, but not so great for oily skin.
5. Solid to cream compacts are not easy to apply and not good for oily skin.
6. Cream to powder formulas give a matte finish without the hassle of applying powder after foundation, but are not good for dry skin, as they accentuate wrinkles.

POWDER. Finishing powders come in two basic forms, pressed or loose. Deciding which powder to use depends on the look you want to achieve. Loose powders tend to give a lighter finish, but application tends to be messy. Pressed powders create a matte, finished look.

EYE SHADOW. The colors available for eye shadows are unlimited. Eye shadow should be worn to enhance the eye, not to color around it. Color on the face should concentrate on the cheeks and lips. Avoid colored eye shadows in blue, violet, green, or red as well as pastel colors. These will add unnecessary color and won't define the eye. Eye shadows that are too shiny, too sheer, or come in difficult-to-use application sets should also be avoided. Experts advise using neutral colors like tan, beige, brown, sable, chestnut, camel, mahogany,

> "You'd be surprised how much it costs to look this cheap."
>
> DOLLY PARTON

hazel, gray, charcoal, slate, mauve, and plum. If you are going to wear a set of eye colors, make sure it is wearable with different outfits, and not just limited to one blouse. Where to put color on the eyelids is equally personal. The general rule is: the lighter color goes all over the eyelid, from the lashes to the eyebrow, and a deeper color goes along the crease and to the back corner of the eye. A highlighter along the brow is optional, but don't make the color too light or eyes will look puffy.

EYELINER. It is best to stick to brown or black when lining the eyes. Liquid liners will give a more dramatic effect, but should only be used to line the lid for evening; in daytime they look too harsh. Thin pencils can be used to create soft or dramatic lines, depending on application technique. Automatic pencils sharpen themselves. Purchasing the right shade of brown or black is personal. If you are going to experiment with colored eye pencils, use caution. Avoid lining eyes in anything neon—unless, of course, it's Halloween.

MASCARA. Standard colors work. Brown and black go a long way. Think twice—or maybe three times—about any other color. Note: Waterproof mascaras do not stay on longer than water-soluble mascaras. Waterproof mascaras are difficult to take off at night, and will pull eyelashes and the skin around the eyes. Water-soluble mascaras will provide the same coverage, but are easier to remove.

BLUSH. Every skin type looks best in colors that are neither too bright nor too pale. Rose, pink, mauve, plum, and coral are good colors to choose from. You can also choose beiges or tans, but these might not give you the intensity of color you may need.

LIPSTICK. The range of colors available is almost as amazing as the names that go along with them. Experiment with different colors to find the ones you like best. Often magazines advise all people with X-color eyes and Y-color skin to use Z-color lipstick. While this advice may prove helpful, try on any lip color before purchasing. Avoid lipsticks that are too shiny or glossy because they are more likely to come off; shiny, luminous, and pearlescent lipsticks tend to turn white after application. Don't feel threatened by the language used to describe lipsticks. The list of terms is endless and confusing. Just keep in mind two basic kinds: matte lipsticks do not shine, give little moisture to the lips, and claim to stay on longer; sheer lipsticks are more translucent and give the lips surface color.

APPLICATION. No magazine, book, friend, or cosmetic salesperson should dictate how much makeup you choose to apply. We recommend a certain amount of makeup that we feel best enhances one's face. This is our opinion—nothing more, nothing less—take it or leave it.

1. FOUNDATION: Never extend foundation onto the neck. Start by taking a makeup wedge (or use your fingers) to smudge and thin foundation all over the face—this will help in areas around the eyes and nose. If you want to dilute the foundation for lighter coverage, blend in some moisturizer or water. Conversely, use a cotton ball for application if you need heavier coverage.

2. CONCEALERS: Keep in mind what you are trying to hide when you apply concealer. Pimples should be covered with concealer before foundation is applied. Under-eye circles should be covered after foundation goes on, so you know how much concealer you need.

TO APPLY CONCEALER: Place three dots, starting from the inside corner of the eye and ending where the lower lashes end. Don't place concealer too far out near the top of the cheek. Repeat the same process on the upper eyelid to create a balance. Then gently use the tips of your fingertips to blend.

3. POWDER: Powder is used to hold the foundation and concealer in place. It gives the effect of a finished look, hence the name "finishing powder." When applying powder, we recommend you use a makeup puff or pad instead of a brush. Too much powder can make the face look cakey and chalky, so use it sparingly. Note: There is a tendency for older women to overuse powder to cover fine lines and wrinkles. Powder seeps into the cracks; if too much is applied, lines of the face will be accentuated instead of covered.

4. EYE SHADOW: Avoid using the sponge-tip applicators that are included in your compact. They layer the eye shadow, making it look cakey and causing it to flake. Use eye-shadow brushes instead.

5. EYELINER: Eyeliners give definition to the eye, and give the illusion of bigger, more pronounced eyes. The trick to application is not to draw a straight line underneath the lashes, but instead to carefully smudge color beneath the eye so that you won't see the line, but rather the effect. Tip: Apply a bit of eye powder over the eye pencil to make the line look less severe. If your eyes are too close, start the eyeliner halfway under the lid, instead of extending fully to the inner corner. Lining the eye on top of the lid will create a more dramatic effect. Whether you choose a liquid eyeliner or a pencil, be careful not to overdo it. Makeup, after all, is supposed to enhance your face—not to stand alone as artwork. If you look in the mirror and see only the eyeliner and the exact line it creates, you know you have overdone it. To avoid eyeliner smudge, use concealers and moisturizers that are oil-free. The fine lines under your eyes will absorb the eye pencil no matter how careful you are, so some smudge will occur.

6. EYEBROWS: Of all the makeup faux pas, nothing can make the face more artificial or dated than improper eyebrow-filling. If you use an eyebrow pencil, don't just draw a line to extend the length of the brow. Natural eyebrows are made up of a group of hairs that create a line. Some eyebrow pencils come with a brush at one end. Use this tool to brush through the line to create a fuller brow. Eyebrow powders and eye shadows that match the brow color don't work as well as pencils. Brow gels are another option. They are similar to mascara brushes, and make the brow look thicker.

7. LIP LINERS: Lip liners work wonders for women who have a hard time putting on their lipstick. Otherwise they are completely optional. Lip liners claim to stop lipsticks from bleeding and give the lips a more defined look. If you like to use them, fine. If you never have used them and don't have a problem putting lipstick on, skip it. Note: Unless you want your lips to look somewhat two-toned, lip liners should either match the natural color of your lips or your lipstick.

8. LIPSTICK: The general rule for application is to line your bottom lip, then rub the upper lip and bottom lip together. Blot your mouth on a piece of tissue to remove any excess, then place some powder over the lips to keep lipstick in place.

9. MASCARA: Leave mascara application to the very end. For best results, curl lashes with an eyelash curler. An eyelash curler is an amazing little gadget, takes a second to use, and makes the eyes look more open. If mascara clumps, think about purchasing a new one.

REMOVING MAKEUP STAINS. Rub stain in shampoo, dishwashing detergent, or non-oil-based makeup remover. Wash as usual.

Makeup Tools

There are some makeup tools that are worth the extra money. The best makeup will not look good if it is not applied correctly, and certain tools are must-haves. They are: a great blush brush, an eye-shadow brush, an eyelash curler, tweezers, lash and brow tool, and a good eyeliner sharpener. All other makeup tools are optional.

Female Facial Hair

WAXING. Waxing on your own is a potentially painful process. The wax must be the right temperature, and your hand must have no mercy. Go to a professional. They will have special creams to put on after waxing is completed which will reduce any redness or irritation.

> "The mirror usually reflects only the way others see us, the way we are expected to behave, forced to behave—hardly what we really are."
>
> **LUIGI PIRANDELLO**

BLEACHING. Best for upper-lip hair, or facial hair. Jolen is the best product to use; however, make sure to follow the instructions so as not to put too much bleach in the mixture. Don't leave the cream on for too long, or irritation may occur, leaving you with little red bumps. Do a patch test on your arm before bleaching to make sure your skin doesn't have a reaction to the product. If redness does occur, rinse your face with cool water, and apply a moisturizing cream to relieve any burning feeling.

CHEMICAL DEPILATORIES. If you can find a depilatory with a reasonable odor that you can leave on for ten to fifteen minutes, this method works well. Caution: Spot-check the product first to make sure your skin does not react adversely to it.

ELECTROLYSIS. The only proven method of hair removal. Afterward, tiny red bumps may occur, but there is nothing you can do to treat them. Wait it out.

HOW TO GROW OUT OVERPLUCKED EYEBROWS. Overplucked eyebrows can take up to three to six weeks to grow back. If you've been overplucking for years to compensate for a tweezing that went awry, some hairs may never grow back. You can make eyebrows fuller by using an eye shadow that matches your natural hair color. Apply it with a fine, stiff eyeliner brush, or an eyebrow pencil. Use small strokes around and underneath the existing brow, and blend with a small toothbrush. To make this brow last, brush some translucent powder over the entire area.

HELPFUL TWEEZING TIPS:
1. A good time to tweeze is after the shower. Since skin is softer then, tweezing will be less painful.
2. Only tweeze in daylight so you can see what you're doing and avoid the morning-after shock from what you did the night before.
3. After you tweeze two to three hairs from one brow, make sure to do the same to the other brow. Before you continue, check to make sure brows are symmetrical.

4. Never pluck the hairs above the brow! Doing so will distort the natural line of the brow.
5. Never tweeze when the phone is ringing, the dog needs to be walked, you've just done your taxes, or you've just drunk five cups of coffee.
6. If you take a pencil and hold it vertically, placing it right beside your nose, the point where the pencil meets the eyebrow is where your brow should start.

Male Facial Hair

SHAVING. While the cosmetic industry would like for us to believe that there exists a product that prepares the beard for the onslaught of shaving cream, a little moisturizer or vegetable oil will do just fine and save you a lot of money. Timing counts when it comes to getting a close shave. After you shower, your pores are open and your beard is wet, making it a prime time to apply shaving cream. Pick the shaving cream you like best. Generally, there is little difference among the widely available brands. Keep in mind that shaving foams must be left in place for a least one minute so they can soak into the beard. Creams and lotions work faster. Rinse your razor under the hottest water possible. Begin with the cheeks, then under your lower lip, and finish with the chin and upper lip. When rinsing, splash the face with warm water repeatedly to make sure all the shaving cream and dirt are removed. If you don't get a smooth shave the first time, do it again. Don't shave against the hair growth; this will result in irritation and rash. After shaving, apply a toner and a moisturizer with sunscreen. A toner will clean off the debris left from shaving, and will close the pores. If you don't want to use a toner, you can splash your face with cold water to get the same effect. A moisturizer or aftershave lotion will soothe the skin, prevent irritation, and protect your face throughout the day. If you never use shaving cream and it has worked well for you, by all means continue your own ritual.

SHAVING BLACK SKIN. Ingrown hairs are particularly prevalent in black men or men of Mediterranean origin because the hair texture is curly and coarse. When hair is shaved it may curl back and grow inward, causing painful boils. To avoid ingrown hairs, take a clean toothbrush and massage the face in circular motions to lift hairs away from the beard. Soak your razor in alcohol for fifteen minutes. During this time, take a sewing needle that has been sterilized in alcohol and gently lift hairs that aren't too far under the skin. With a warm washcloth, soak your skin for five minutes to allow hairs to swell and lift even more, and lather with a shaving cream for sensitive skin. Shave in the direction of the hair growth. Afterward apply a toner and a moisturizer with a sunscreen.

> ## "A nose that can see is worth two that can sniff."
>
> **EUGÈNE IONESCO**

MUSTACHES AND BEARDS. Mustaches and beards are to men as eyebrows and hair are to women: both can enhance the shape of the face. Facial hair must suit an individual's facial features, and should be kept trimmed and neatly groomed. If you're not willing to take care of your facial hair, don't bother growing it—nothing is more unsightly than an overgrown beard or mustache. Patience is another prerequisite for growing facial hair. Hair growth will vary from person to person. It is best to start growing a beard while you're on vacation because the initial scruffiness might not be appropriate for work. Wait to style your beard or mustache until it has filled in. Don't be surprised if your facial hair grows in a different color than your hair. If the facial hair color is too different or dramatic, talk to your hairdresser about dying and coloring possibilities. The shape of your face should dictate what kind of beard or mustache you grow. Here are some guidelines: Nose shape—Large noses should have an equally large mustache, which will help to balance the nose. Small noses should stay away from the Groucho Marx look. Shape of your face—If your face is thin or narrow, a full short beard and mustache will give the illusion of a fuller face. If your face is elongated, avoid long beards—they will appear to drag your face downward still more. If your face is full, equally full beards and mustaches suit you well.

CAMOUFLAGE. A beard will hide full cheeks, signs that you have gained weight, or a weak chin. Camouflaging a weak chin with a beard will be effective only if it is grown from ear to ear. Hair on the chin alone will make a weak chin more pronounced.

RATIO OF HAIR TO FACIAL HAIR FACTOR. Bald men should not overcompensate by growing very full beards and mustaches, unless you intend to look like ZZ Top. If the hair on your head is trimmed short, your facial hair should also be short; longer facial hair looks good with a full head of hair. In short, facial hair should mimic the cut and style of one's hair. Ask your hairdresser for recommendations if you are unsure.

TRIMMING BEARDS AND MUS-TACHES. You should trim your beard and/or mustache at least once a week. The easiest way is to comb through the hair, lifting it up and cutting across with a pair of scissors or an electric razor. Then brush the hair in the direction you want it to go. Remember to shave the areas around your facial hair to keep your beard and mustache looking trim. If you are a first-time facial-hair owner, you might want to go to your hairdresser for advice to avoid potential problems.

CLEANING. Use a gentle shampoo every day. Facial hair can be coarser than the hair on your head, so applying conditioner regularly will help to maintain softness. Don't neglect to provide a skin-care regime for the skin under your beard or mustache.

"She gave me a smile I could feel in my hip pocket."

RAYMOND CHANDLER

Eyes

STYES. Styes are an infection caused by bacteria trapped in the eye. A sty usually appears in the corner of the eye, and looks like a small boil that secretes a yellow pus at the surface. To treat it, get eyedrops of saline solution or boric acid from any pharmacy. Your pharmacist will advise you on how many drops should be placed in the eye. Styes are contagious, so avoid touching or placing any contact on the sty while it is healing. Recovery time is ten days to two weeks.

PINK EYE. If your eye is crusty, hard to open, itchy, and swollen, you probably have pink eye. See an optometrist for treatment.

SURGERY VS. GLASSES. Wearing eyeglasses or contacts may be your best bet to correct nearsightedness. Over the past fifteen years, out of the one million Americans who have undergone radial keratomy—surgery to correct nearsightedness—one-fifth of the patients were overcorrected by the surgery and as a result became farsighted. Three percent of these people had worse vision after their operations. So before going under the knife, make sure your doctor is a true corneal specialist or you'll be replacing the glasses you wore to the movies with glasses you need for reading.

EYELASH REMOVAL. Being blessed with long eyelashes sometimes causes temporary discomfort. When an eyelash gets stuck in the eye, fold the upper lid over the lower lid and move the eyeball around so the eyelash falls out of the corner of the eye.

STARRY-EYED. Have you ever wondered why sometimes you see stars? Apparently, when the eye's natural cleaning fluid replenishes itself, the process temporarily floods the eye, thus causing you to see stars.

CHOOSING THE RIGHT CONTACT LENSES. Now that contact lenses are available for most vision problems (there are even bifocal contacts), the most important factor in choosing lenses is comfort vs. health. Hard contact lenses, while not as comfortable as soft, actually are healthier, because they allow better circulation of oxygen to the eyes. (Soft lenses should be replaced every other week. Contaminants and protein deposits from tears build up even with daily cleaning.) The health differences between the two aren't great, but extended-wear lenses are comfortable. Wearing lenses around the clock can cause sight-threatening conditions such as infections and corneal ulcers because the eye is being deprived of oxygen. Infrequent cleaning also means that the eye is constantly exposed to contaminants that accumulate on the lens. If you like the comfort of extended-wear lenses, consider using them like daily wear hard lenses. Note: Eye care should include a yearly checkup by an optometrist.

Nose

NOSEBLEEDS. Often caused by winter's dry indoor air, nosebleeds occur when blood vessels rupture close to the surface on the front part of the nasal linings. Don't panic: nosebleeds look more serious than they really are. Sit or lie down with the head elevated higher than the level of the heart. Then pinch the soft parts of the nose together with your thumb and two fingers, using a tissue or cloth, and exert pressure firmly toward the face for five minutes. If bleeding persists, it could be a sign that blood is coming deep from within the nose, with blood flowing down the throat. In that unlikely situation, treatment is best left to a doctor.

SPIDER NEVI. Spider nevi—better known as broken nose-capillaries—are veins that become engorged and show through the skin's surface, appearing as tiny bluish or red lines. This condition is benign and should not cause worry. The formation of the lines is thought to be of genetic or developmental origin. Alcoholism can contribute to this condition, since it breaks down the skin's tissue. Long-term exposure to the sun without protection is another external cause. The reason these lines are more pronounced in older people is related to decreasing elasticity, reduction of fat, and thinning of the skin as a result of the aging process. Cosmetic surgery can be performed to remove spider nevi, and has a high rate of success.

RED NOSE. These large raised spots on the nose are caused by an engorgement of the blood vessels which form tumorlike red spots on the outer part of the nose. After puberty these spots will become more pronounced as the skin changes. People who are genetically predisposed to getting them should expect the spots to appear as they age.

COLDS. **WHAT ARE THEY?** An infection of the upper respiratory system, caused by a common virus that is incurable, uncomfortable, and relatively harmless.
HOW YOU GET THEM. Either by standing close enough to an infected person to breathe in the live virus from coughs and sneezes, or by touching your eyes, nose, or mouth to a virus-laden surface.
HOW YOU DON'T GET THEM. Wet feet. Kissing (well, you can get a cold from kissing an infected partner, but for unknown reasons it only happens 10 percent of the time).
HOW LONG THEY LAST. Symptoms arrive within ten to twelve hours of exposure, and take about six or seven days to go away.

WHY YOUR NOSE RUNS. Because irritated blood vessels in the nose begin to leak plasma. This is thought to be a defensive maneuver to irrigate and cleanse infected cells.
WHY YOU SNEEZE AND COUGH. Sneezing results when the tiny hairs lining the nasal cavity are overwhelmed by mucus and can't sweep out foreign particles on their own; it's the difference between getting mud off your hands with a trickle of water from the tap and flooding it away with a garden hose. The coughing reflex switches on to aid the body in getting rid of all the excess fluid produced by the nose, throat, and blood vessels.
HOW YOU CAN PREVENT THEM. You can't. But repeated studies show that megadoses of vitamin C during the cold and flu season can greatly reduce their severity.
WHY YOU SHOULD LISTEN TO YOUR MOTHER. (a) Chicken soup works, especially spicy chicken soup, because the spice acts as an expectorant. It's important to drink plenty of liquids when you have a cold, because you lose moisture when you spend a lot of time breathing through your mouth, and you can easily worsen your symptoms; and (b) Chicken contains a natural amino acid called cystine. Cystine is chemically similar to a drug called acetylcysteine, which doctors prescribe for patients with bronchitis and respiratory infections.

NOSE RINGS. To avoid infection, be sure to wipe both the ring and your nose with alcohol.

Ears

EARWAX: Earwax is the ear's way of lubricating the skin of the ear canal. It serves to repel water and to prevent bacteria from reaching the eardrum. Often referred to as potato sacs, a certain amount of earwax is normal. If your earwax builds up too much, a careful cleaning with a cotton swab will remove the excess. However, be careful not to swab too deeply into the ear canal. If the buildup makes it difficult to hear, don't use a cotton swab to clear the ear canal. Instead, flush the ear canal with warm water to melt the wax and allow it to fall out naturally.

NOISE: Yes, your mother was right: loud noise can hurt your ears. After three decades of rock and roll, musicians and fans alike have come back to report that the loud, constant noise to their ears has left them with severely damaged hearing. And there is no way to restore life to dead nerve endings; the damage is permanent. Why? Cilia, the hairs in the ear that change sound waves into nerve impulses, weren't designed to shake as hard as they do when exposed to a loud sound. How loud does it have to be? Any sound that causes you to shout over background noise to make yourself heard, makes your ears ring, causes pain, or makes you slightly deaf for several hours after exposure, is potentially damaging. Experts agree that continual exposure to more than 85 decibels may become dangerous. If you are exposed to loud noises every now and then—like an occasional

"Any man over 30 with long hair looks like his mother."

ORSON WELLES

concert—chances are you won't be significantly affected. However, the longer you are exposed to a loud noise, the more damaging it will be. Cilia have no pain cells, so if you are damaging your ears, you probably won't feel it. Wear protective earplugs if you are around loud noises; people who work in factories, construction, and the music business should be especially careful. Blasting your favorite tunes through your Walkman can also be potentially damaging. Hearing loss develops over a period of time. If you have ringing in your ears, or have trouble understanding people at parties where there is background noise, it may be just a sign of wax buildup or an infection, but it could be the first sign of permanent hearing loss. Consult your doctor or an ear specialist if the problem persists.

SWIMMER'S EAR. An inflammation of the lining of the ear canal that occurs when the ear is exposed to excess water. Too much water or moisture in the ear washes away the ear's waxy protective coating, which contains antibacterial materials. Dead skin cells gather in the ear canal and create a nesting ground for bacteria to grow and infect the ear. The first symptoms are pain around the earlobes, which becomes noticeable when you chew or lie on your side. How do you prevent it? Wear earplugs when swimming, thoroughly dry the ears after bathing or swimming, and don't let wet, long hair hang over the ears. How do you know you have it? The ear may feel blocked, or itch. In later stages, the ear canal will become swollen, and sometimes will swell shut. A runny, milky liquid might drain out of the ear, and the ear will be painful, especially to the touch. How do you treat it? Keep the ears dry for at least three days, or as much as a week, depending on the severity. Over-the-counter eardrops or antibiotics may be prescribed. If pain continues, and milky drainage starts, see a doctor.

POPPING. Most of us have experienced an uncomfortable, stuffed-up, blocked feeling in our ears, either in an airplane, in a car going up an elevation, or when we have a cold. Why this occurs has to do with the ear equalizing itself with the air pressure on both sides of the eardrum. When the air pressure is not equal, the ear feels blocked. How do you unblock your ears? Chewing gum or sucking on a candy will induce swallowing, which opens the air passage of the ear called the Eustachian tube. Yawning is an even better activator of this muscle. If this doesn't work, pinch your nostrils shut, and then take a mouthful of air. Using your cheek and throat muscles, force the air into the back of your nose as if you were trying to blow your thumb and fingers off your nostrils. When you hear a loud pop in your ears, you

have succeeded. You may have to repeat this several times. Babies cannot pop their ears by themselves, so it is best to have them suck on a bottle or pacifier during an airplane descent. Tips: Don't use your chest or abdomen to create the force to inflate your ears. The proper technique involves only pressure created by your cheek and throat muscles. If you have a cold, a sinus infection, an allergy attack, or have recently undergone ear surgery, it is best to postpone air travel.

ALFRED E. NEWMAN EARS. Each year more than 10,000 Americans undergo otoplasty, otherwise known as "pinning back" the ears. And that's exactly what the procedure is: permanent stitches are placed in the back of the ear to anchor them to the head. Ideally, the operation is performed when a child is five or six.

EARLOBE DROOP. Some of us, as we age, find that our earlobes stick out, don't match, or sag. In another extremely simple procedure, a plastic surgeon can trim excess flesh to make the lobes more symmetrical or less droopy; or, a well-placed stitch can hold down lobes that stick out.

BIG EARS. They're much harder to correct. Here the ear is made smaller by cutting away a section in the middle, as if removing a slice of pie, and then the edges of the remaining tissue are rejoined.

Lips

CANKER SORES. Ulcerous sores on the lips may have come from the herpes simplex virus, or a variety of other causes. If they're herpes sores, they go away in a few days without treatment. (The antiviral drug acyclovir is sometimes prescribed.) But if you find they occur repeatedly, try taking folic acid and B_{12} supplements; sometimes these sores result from deficiencies of these two vitamins.

CHAPPED LIPS. Vaseline or Chap Stick is the best and cheapest remedy for chapped lips; Elizabeth Arden's Eight Hour Cream is a more

expensive, but highly effective lubricant. If you are going to be in the sun, however, use a sun-protective lip balm.

TO REMOVE LIPSTICK STAINS. Several options: Non-oil-based makeup remover, a non-gel toothpaste, dry-cleaning solvent—or a piece of mushy white bread (Wonder Bread works well). After applying, wash as usual. If color remains, try soaking in water and ammonia.

"The only thing that can stop hair falling is the floor."

WILL ROGERS

Teeth

PROBLEMS WITH BLEACHING. Over-the-counter hydrogen peroxide products may temporarily damage the mouth's soft tissues and the pulp of teeth. Researchers are also looking into irreversible cell changes that may cause cancer.

DENTURES. When choosing dentures, make sure the fit is comfortable—there should be no abrasion of the gum or bone tissue. Dentures should also have a good relationship with the lip. Make sure to smile to see how much tooth and gum you want to show. Often people assume that their dentures are going to feel like their original teeth. Check in the mirror before you leave the dentist's office. Finally, you should test the color of the dentures in real daylight, not the artificial light often found in dentists' offices. The two common kinds of dentures are porcelain, which gives a more realistic appearance, and acrylic, which gives a slightly more bluish white cast.

SENSITIVE TEETH. If you experience a burning, numbing sensation in your teeth when you drink coffee or eat ice cream, you know how painful this problem can be. Sensitive teeth actually have nothing at all to do with the teeth themselves. The problem occurs when there is a loss of gum tissue and the roots of the teeth are exposed to the air, making that part of the teeth hypersensitive to extremes of hot or cold. Treatment? Use a toothpaste especially designed for sensitive teeth, which helps coat the sensitive area. The best way to prevent the condition is daily flossing and gentle brushing of the gums. See a dentist if the problem persists.

GUM DISEASE. Gum disease is an infection which is caused by plaque, the bacterial film that coats the teeth. If unremoved by proper brushing and flossing, plaque produces toxins that can irritate the gums. In the early stages, gum disease can be reversed. In later phases, called periodontitis, the bone and tissue that support teeth may be affected, causing tooth loss.
WARNING SIGNS. Gums that are swollen, red, bleed (when you brush or floss), or recede to the root of the tooth are early signs of gum disease. In advanced cases, loose teeth, persistent bad breath, or pus between the gums or teeth are indications that an immediate trip to the dentist's is needed.
PREVENTION. Brush at least twice a day, floss, and use Stimu-Dent sticks (Johnson & Johnson) to reach stubborn plaque. See a dentist twice a year for proper cleaning to remove hardened plaque, called tartar, or when problems first appear. If left untreated, some gum diseases may require surgery.

BAD BREATH. All of us have dragon breath at some time—usually the first thing in the morning, when our saliva flow has decreased overnight, leaving aromatic bacteria to nibble at stray food particles left in the mouth from last night's dinner. In most cases, brushing the teeth and tongue helps. So does eating some fresh parsley—the chlorophyll works on the odors. What doesn't work too well is mouthwash: it masks the odor for a little while, but it does not kill the bacteria that cause bad breath. In fact, the alcohol in some mouthwashes can dry out the mouth, ultimately making breath worse.

Hair

You can't change your hair type. No product will make curly hair straight or straight hair curly unless you opt for a chemical process. But whatever your hair type, the products you use on your hair can make a difference to a certain extent. Does this mean that you must buy the most expensive products available, or those that your hairdresser swears by? Probably not. Most shampoos and conditioners have similiar formulas, much like skin-care products, and pricy products are no guarantee of effectiveness. However, if you find something that works well on your hair, stick with it. Part of finding good hair-care products involves experimentation. If you spend the night at a friend's house, using an unfamiliar shampoo or conditioner the next morning can introduce you to a new product that works for you. Here are some general guidelines for different hair types, and what types of products work best.

DRY HAIR. Coarse and curly hair tends to get dry. If left alone, hair has the potential to be unruly and wild, so the best products to use are heavier, creamier formulas that decrease volume and add moisture. Blow-drying hair will make dry hair look frizzy. If you must, use a diffuser and scrunch curls into place. It is not necessary to shampoo dry hair daily. Though they clean the hair, shampoos tend to strip oils and moisture from the scalp that dry hair needs. Curly hair looks best when shampooed two to three times a week. You might notice that on the days you don't shampoo, your hair will look better. Conditioning is a key step in managing curly hair. There are many good conditioners on the market designed for curly hair. Manufacturers often distribute sample packets of their products; play around. Deep-conditioning once or twice every two weeks is also helpful for keeping dry hair in condition. Silicone sprays and serums, and polishing sprays, are great new styling tools that help defrizz curly hair, smooth the hair cuticle, and enhance shine.

> "I wouldn't mind being the last man on earth—just to see if all those girls were telling me the truth."
>
> **RONNIE SHAKES**

OILY HAIR. Limp, fine, and thin hair tends to get oily. Shampooing regularly with a heavier, more concentrated shampoo will draw extra oil out from the scalp and hair shaft. Oily hair does not need to be conditioned since the hair naturally lubricates itself. However, to avoid tangles and snarls after shampooing, it is helpful to run a light conditioner through the hair. To add body, there are products such as mousse, root volumizers, and volumizers which make fine hair thicker and heavier.

NORMAL HAIR. Hair that maintains style or curl easily is defined as normal. Shampooing with a moisturizing shampoo and conditioner will maintain healthy hair. To help boost the effect of a curling iron or rollers, use a setting spray which will lock hair into the desired shape. There are heat-activated sprays which will respond to the heat of a curling iron or rollers to help hair that is on the coarser side of normal. To create a smoother look, use a strong gel that will hold hair in a desired style. For the wet look, use a water-based gel without a blow-dryer. For a softer look, use a blow-dryer and a brush. Sculpting lotion, creams, or spray gels all work well on normal hair to help create the style you desire.

SPLIT ENDS. When there is a lack of moisture at the ends of the hair, or when hair is overbrushed or overdried, the ends of the hair will simply break off and split. Split ends are a good sign that a haircut or trim is overdue. To prevent split ends, use gentle brushes, and wide-tooth combs to distribute the scalp's oil to hair ends. Try not to pull too hard on your hair. Don't stretch or pull your hair. If you must use a blow-dryer, keep it on a medium or cool setting. Lastly, products with silicone in them help to bond split ends until you can make an appointment at the hairdresser's.

TIPS AND MYTHS:

1. Just because the hair-deity came up with three hair types doesn't mean your hair fits perfectly into one category. Some days your hair may be dry; other days it might be oily. Somehow, bad-hair days seem to arrive on important occasions. You know your hair best— what it needs, and what makes it look good. If a hairdresser promises that he will make your curly hair stay straight, it is best to politely excuse yourself. Once you accept your hair type and experiment with different products to see which ones work, you'll be on your way to becoming your own hair expert.

2. When using a hair dryer, it is best to use a styling product to protect hair from becoming dry.

3. Sun damages hair, just as it damages skin if not protected. When going to the beach, or exposing hair to the sun for a prolonged period of time, use a UVA/UVB protective hair product.

4. When hair is wet, putting it in a tight ponytail might cause breakage as hair dries and expands. After a shower, wait 15 minutes before using a tight elastic to pull hair back.

5. It is not true that ponytails cause hair to fall out. However, hair that is always in a tight ponytail, or is pulled back, might be more prone to breakage.

6. Before perming or coloring your hair, make sure it's in good condition. Although many advances have been made in safer methods, you will get the best results if your hair is in good condition before it's treated.

7. Myth: Hair needs to be cut every eight weeks. Fact: Hair should be cut when you feel it should be cut.

8. After a shower, use a wide-tooth comb to brush hair out. Don't use a fine-tooth comb, or a brush with too many bristles. Both make hair more prone to breakage.

FACTS:

1. The number of times the average American man washes his hair during his lifetime: 18,325. The number of times the average American woman washes her hair: 15,696.

2. In Fiji, touching a woman's hair is as taboo as reaching out and touching the genitals of a stranger would be in our culture.

3. The most promising treatments for hair loss are yet to come: researchers are working to develop drugs that modify the hormonal processes which influence male pattern baldness.

Color

HENNA. **WHAT IS IT?** Henna is a natural vegetable dye used for thousands of years in India, the Middle East, and North Africa to dye hair various shades of red. How it works depends on your hair type, the type of henna used (different countries produce different kinds), the color of your hair, the amount of time it is left on the hair, and other herbs that are used. When using it for the first time, test it on a strand of hair. The best way is to use hair left on your comb or brush. If the treatments are used periodically, the results will be better. For people who are beginning to go gray, henna works wonders.

HOW TO USE IT? By mixing it with boiling water so it turns into a creamy solution, and then applying it to the hair under a dryer. To tone down the red, you can use a strong tea instead of boiling water. You can soften or intensify the color by halving or doubling the amount of herbs, such as walnut husks or artichoke leaves. Ask your herbalist for more information.

GROWING IT OUT. Wait as long as you can before seeing the hairdresser. The biggest mistake people make is taking too much off, too often. Hair should be trimmed a quarter of an inch every eight to nine weeks. Layers should be trimmed only a little bit—an eighth of an inch.

TO COLOR OR NOT TO COLOR. Be honest with yourself about your commitment to the change you're making. Radical change may require radical amounts of upkeep. Ask your colorist to discuss options with you, and LISTEN CAREFULLY to what he/she tells you is and is not feasible. Some kinds of very coarse, curly, gray hair, for example, are extremely resistant to coverage. And if your hair has already been colored and/or damaged, it may take several visits to get the results you want. Do not assume you have to get blonder as we get older. Blonding-with-the-years is one hair tradition that most colorists are trying to banish: hair color should be dictated by complexion, not age. Warming hair tones, not lightening them, should be the goal.

Skin

RASHES. A rash is often the first sign that something is going wrong inside our bodies. Anything and everything can cause a rash— stress, infection, illness, food, drugs, and fever are common instigators. Most rashes do not need any medical treatment, and will go away by themselves; razor burn would fit under this category. But if a rash is painful, takes longer than one day to go away, or comes on suddenly, it is best to consult a dermatologist. Hives often look worse than they really are. An easily treatable rash, hives look like large red welts, and can be very painful and itchy. Stress, fever, or infection are likely candidates for bringing them on. An over-the-counter antihistamine, such as Benadryl, is recommended for treatment. If hives continue to appear regularly, see a dermatologist.

BASAL-CELL CANCER. The least dangerous skin cancer, and by far the most common. They usually appear on sites exposed to the sun, but don't spread. Often, they are pinkish, solid, smooth-surfaced, or pitted nodules that grow slowly and bleed easily.

SQUAMOUS-CELL CANCER. These skin growths are more serious than basal-cell cancer because they can spread to distant sites. They often appear as sores that won't heal, or as crusted, heaped-up nodules. More serious than basal-cell cancer, the tumors can spread to distant sites such as lymph nodes or internal organs. They may develop from solar keratoses, burn sites, or skin damaged by radiation.

MELANOMA. Potentially deadly, and fortunately uncommon. Look for a mole with (a) asymmetry (if you drew a line down the middle of a melanoma, one half would look different from the other); (b) an uneven or blurry border; and (c) a variety of colors (most normal moles are brownish, but a melanoma has a mixture of various shades and colors, including black, brown, red, tan, and white). Note: The secret to treating all skin cancers successfully is to detect them early.

Scrub

SALT SCRUBS. Particularly helpful in relaxing tired muscles and joints; gets rid of dull, dead skin cells. Just think of your body as the rim of a margarita glass, and you get the idea.

HYDROTHERAPY AND BODY BUFFS. Hydrotherapy—basically, the buffeting of the body with high-powered streams of water—won't get rid of bodily "toxins" or reduce cellulite. But the massage and rubdown, often preceded by oils rubbed into the skin, can make you feel new and shiny.

Female Breast

HOW TO DO A BREAST SELF-EXAMINATION Stand in the shower and lift your right arm above your head. Soap your breast so that your fingers slide easily over it. With your left hand, work your fingertips lightly but firmly down your breast in vertical strips, starting from the top and working down toward the bottom. Feel for any bumps or lumps that you haven't felt previously. While the vast majority of breast lumps are non-malignant, if you find one, make

an appointment with your doctor immediately; most researchers today believe the earlier breast cancer is detected, the higher the rate of cure. Breasts should be examined right after your period has ended, when they are less swollen.

MAKING BREASTS FIRMER. Breast tissue is mostly fat, and exercise is not going to change your breast size. But by exercising the muscles underneath the breast, large breasts will look firmer and sit higher on the chest, while those with small breasts can achieve something approaching cleavage. These exercises utilize free weights, but machines can also be used. Try to perform at least one of them between six and twelve repetitions each set, and two to three sets per exercise, twice a week, gradually upping the poundage on the free weights as you gain strength.
1. Dumbbell flys: Lie back on a flat bench with your feet touching the floor. With a dumbbell in each hand, extend your arms to a position directly over your chest, with the palms of your hands pointing in. Bend your elbows slightly and slowly lower your arms out to the sides as low as possible. Then push the weights back up, following the same path you used to lower them.
2. Barbell bench press: Lie back on a flat exercise bench and take a grip on the bar that's slightly wider than your shoulders. Have a spotter lift the bar off the rack for you. Move the bar into a straight-arm position directly above your chest. Then slowly lower the bar to your chest, about midway between your breasts and shoulder line. Now slowly press back up to the straight-arm position, with your elbows locked. Don't let the bar bounce off your chest after the lowering phase of the exercise. Bouncing could injure your chest and rib cage. Nor should you arch your back during the lift; that action could put pressure on your spine. Keep your feet flat on the floor and your back pressed close to the bench.

BRAS FOR EXERCISING. A good bra when exercising will eliminate the painful bouncing of breasts. Look for heavy support no matter how large or small your breast size. Exercise bras should fit a bit snugger than your everyday bras. Two factors that are important for

comfort are inner-cup sculpting, which keeps breasts from rubbing together, and adjustable straps and back, which enhance fit and make the bra easy to get on and off.

> "They say if you smoke you knock off ten years. But it's the last ten. What do you miss? The drooling years?"
>
> JOHN MENDOZA

BRALESS. Every woman should have the right to go braless. But those of us over a B-cup size rarely feel too comfortable swinging in the breeze; we want to be hip, but we're quietly thinking to ourselves, "Moo." As the years pass, the larger the breast size, the greater the tendency for breasts to be victims of gravity. (This is particularly true of women who have had several children, with concomitant breast swelling during each pregnancy.) The only defense is making sure you invest in the best-quality bra (read: best-supporting bras; underwire is your friend).

BREAST IMPLANTS: SILICONE VS. SALINE. Many women have been returning to their doctors to have their silicone implants removed and saline implants put in their place. However, saline doesn't feel as natural as silicone gel. Gel flows; saline moves fast and can create a waviness in the skin. There's enormous debate on this issue, but doctors believe that unless there's a specific medical problem—for example, the formation of scar tissue which makes breasts harden unnaturally—there's not enough clinical evidence to warrant removal of the silicone implants.

The Back

BACK PAIN. Back pain is caused by a myriad of factors, ranging from overexertion to more serious bone alignment problems. Most back pain is the result of spine-related musculoskeletal problems that are not inflammatory, infectious, or related to abnormal tissue development. Herniated discs, degenerative disc disease, fractures, and other injuries fall into this category. However, back pain may signal serious underlying problems. If it begins unexpectedly (not after you just lifted furniture), it is best to see a doctor immediately to rule out the possibility of other diseases or fractures. Also, if your pain radiates out to other parts of your body such as the buttocks, legs, or arms, if your legs feel numb or weak, or if you lose control of your bladder or bowels, see a physician immediately. A report from the *Journal of the American Medical Association* estimates that 85 percent of people with chronic lower back pain cannot be given a clear diagnosis as to why their pain exists. Doctors think that common back pain may be attributed to degenerative changes or muscle shifts in the back, but they aren't really sure. This uncertainty isn't too comforting for victims of lower back pain. Some things that are known to relieve back pain include: a firm mattress, changing your desk chair, lifting with your legs, not sleeping on your stomach, and not slouching when you stand. (But don't mention these suggestions to any back pain sufferer, particularly if their back is "out" at the time—the response will not be pleasant.) If chronic pain persists, seeing a doctor should be your first step.

CONVENTIONAL TREATMENTS. Chiropractic treatment is based on the theory that a person's well-being is contingent on the relationship between the musculoskeletal and nervous systems (the muscles and the nerves). The theory holds that misalignment of the vertebrae (the back being crooked) can cause pain; thus treatment involves a form of bone-cracking which increases a stiff joint's range of motion and stretches tightened muscles and ligaments. Medical institutions turn their nose up at chiropractic treatment, but those afflicted with back pain see chiropractors twice as often as they see medical doctors. Osteopathy, in layman's terms, is the medical form of chiropractic treatment. Both approaches believe in the muscle-to-nerve relationship, but osteopathic physicians take into account an individual's general health as well. If a chiropractor's quick thrusts and twist movements scare you, osteopathic manipulations might be a better choice.

UNCONVENTIONAL TREATMENTS. There are lots of alternatives in treating back pain that lie outside the border of traditional medicine. The McKenzie Approach centers on the pattern of the back pain, from where it starts to where it goes to what causes it. Therapists who use this approach believe that for every movement or posture that causes back pain, there's an opposite movement or posture that reduces the discomfort. The patient is taught simple exercises that he can perform alone to relieve his pain and help to prevent future problems from erupting. Similarly, the Feldenkrais Method teaches patients how to relax both physically and psychologically by guiding patients through a series of strange positions and movements to make them more aware of the everyday movements which may be causing the pain. Acupuncture is very quickly gaining popularity with American back-pain sufferers. Acupuncture rests on the belief that inside our bodies are energy pathways, called meridians, which connect every organ, every tissue, every cell we have to each other. Illness or back pain is believed to be the result of blockages in this energy flow; thus acupuncturists attempt to relieve back pain by inserting thin needles at various points along the body to free the meridian flow. The Sarno Theory, originated by Dr. John Sarno, holds that a great deal of the pain we feel in life—and nearly all back pain—is manufactured by the subconscious mind to keep our attention away from painful emotions. He believes that back pain is caused by the brain decreasing the amount of oxygen that muscles in the back receive from blood vessels, a protective reaction to repressed anger that we harbor.

QUICK FIXES:

1. Rest. If your back hurts and you can stay in bed for a few days, do it. But don't vegetate for too long. Most clinicians believe too much rest can be detrimental because back muscles will become weak, and inactivity causes the atrophying of muscles. So don't use back pain as an excuse to stay in bed for a week, unless instructed by a doctor to do so.

2. Ice it before you heat it. For the first 48 hours apply ice to sore muscles, and take aspirin, which relieves pain and inflammation.

3. When pain has subsided and you're up and about, start to include strength-training exercises for your back in your exercise regime.

4. Lose weight. Being overweight will not cause back pain, but it will put your back under more stress.

> "The heart has reasons that reason does not understand."
>
> JACQUES BÉNIGNE

MASSAGE. Different kinds of massage work better than others, depending on the degree and acuteness of the pain you experience. Consult your doctor to find out what form of massage would be best for you. The two basic kinds: **1.** Swedish massage, which works on the soft tissue and muscle areas throughout the back. It stimulates the circulation of the lymphatic drainage system, which gets clogged up by lactic acid formed by overexercising. The masseuse uses a range of motions and circular movements to move the sore muscle or joint to its maximum capacity. Athletes, pregnant women, or people who have sore back muscles would all benefit. **2.** Shiatsu is the finger version of acupuncture. Instead of using needles to release the blocked areas of the meridian, the masseuse will use her fingers. Great for people with bladder infections, bone cancer, or ordinary back pain.

Muscles

EXERCISE. **MORE ISN'T NECESSARILY BETTER:** After burning about 3,500 calories a week in exercise (roughly the equivalent of five hours of running), the law of diminishing returns kicks in: health benefits plateau, and significantly more exercise not only may strain joints and ligaments but can also compromise the immune system. Researchers aren't quite sure why, but they suspect it has something to do with the way exercise affects our hormone balance. Epinephrine, a stress hormone that suppresses the immune system, begins to surge in the bloodstream when exertion reaches about 60 percent intensity. When exertion climbs to 75 to 80 percent, stress-induced cortisol also begins to spill into the bloodstream, adding to the overall immunity-suppressing effect.

RELIEF. **RELIEVING SORE MUSCLES:** Overexertion through vigorous exercise is the primary cause of muscle pain. Often neglected is a thorough stretching routine before you begin any physical exercise. Your muscles don't share your sense of urgency about working out—they need to first to wake up. Don't run,

garden, lift, or do any exercise without stretching. If you are exercising in the cold, dress your muscles appropriately; if exercising in hot weather, make sure to drink plenty of fluids to prevent fatigue and injury. Stretching should also be practiced after exercising, when muscles are warm. To relieve muscle pain, the general rule is to put an Ace bandage around the area of discomfort and keep the muscle elevated for 24 to 72 hours. Apply ice for 15 minutes every two hours, and rest as much as possible. After two to three days of rest, soak the muscles in a warm bath. The average time for healing should be about one to two days, during which low-impact exercise will help to prevent further tightening and cramping of the muscles. Even when lifting weights, a 48-hour resting period is needed before working the same muscle group again. If you see or feel a large defect in the muscle, and can't move it normally, consult a physician. Be kind to your muscles and they will be strong for you.

Fat

CELLULITE. We all know what cellulite looks like. If you don't, you are one of the blessed. The dimpled, lumpy fat that may appear anywhere on the lower half of your body, often referred to as "cottage-cheese" skin, is a form of fat that gets trapped in the tissue that anchors the skin and muscle together. Some people are hereditarily predisposed to getting cellulite; others get it because their weight frequently fluctuates, causing their skin to lose its elasticity. The older we get, the more prone we are to develop cellulite, because skin loses its tautness as we age. Women are more likely to have cellulite than men because women gain weight vertically, making room for little pouches of fat to form. Men gain fat horizontally, so their fat gets distributed more evenly. Men's skin is thicker than women's skin, making it less apt to dimple. Enough said. How can we get rid of it? **WORKING OUT:** No matter how hard you exercise, cellulite will not go away if you are prone to getting it. This is not to say that all those leg lifts are going to waste. If you build and tone muscles, the shape of your body will look

better, even if you still have cellulite. It's impossible to get rid of it by using the StairMaster. **COSMETIC CREAMS AND SCRUBBERS:** Some creams will tighten the skin and make it look smoother, but there is not a cream on the market that will break down fatty tissue or eradicate cellulite. Scrubbing or massaging with these products will temporarily improve the skin by increasing circulation and causing skin to swell, but it will not eradicate the cellulite. **OTHER MYTHS:** Caffeine will penetrate the skin, causing cellulite breakdown.

WHAT TO DO: Avoid eating fried foods; avoid repeated weight gain or loss; stop smoking; and stay away from alcohol, sugar, and hot baths. Eat a low-fat diet that includes lots of vegetables and fruits. Limit your intake of dairy products, and get plenty of exercise to help tighten and tone the muscles. Another alternative: Learn to live with it.

Penis

CLEAN. On an uncircumcised man, smegma—the cheesy, odoriferous substance secreted by the sebaceous glands of the penis—can accumulate underneath the foreskin. In order

> # "When my mom found my diaphragm, I told her it was a bathing cap for my cat."
>
> LIZ WINSTON

to clean properly, the man must roll his foreskin back while he's in the shower, wash thoroughly with soap and water (being careful not to get soap into the opening of the urethra—*yowtch!*), and dry carefully with a towel.

TESTICLE CANCER. From adolescence on, men should get into the habit of giving themselves a thorough testicle examination every month to feel for any irregular new lumps. Testicle cancer tends to strike men between the ages of 16 and 33, but older men are also affected, and it is otherwise undetectable. If caught in its early stages, testicle cancer can be treated with a reasonable rate of success.

PROSTATE CANCER. Every man over 50 should see a doctor annually for a rectal exam to check for any abnormalities of the prostate. Black men and those men who have a strong family history of this disease can be given a blood test called PSA, which has recently become available to detect prostate cancer.

YEAST INFECTIONS. If a man has sexual intercourse with a woman who has a yeast infection, he can also become infected and develop a red, splotchy, itchy rash on his penis. It is best to abstain from sexual intercourse while the penis is infected, since intercourse will reinfect the woman. See a doctor for prescriptive medications that will clear the infection.

GENITAL WARTS AND HERPES. Finding either one of these on your penis can be, to say the least, traumatic. Herpes can appear as small water blisters that burn and itch and should be looked at by a doctor. The same goes for genital warts. Most rashes on the penis can be easily treated by prescriptive medications.

BRIEFS VS. BOXERS. The choice of which underwear to wear is a matter of comfort. Tightie-whities give more support, and are best to wear when exercising, running, or doing anything involving bouncing. Boxer shorts give a looser fit, and come in more designs, colors,

and patterns. There is, however, one little note: sperm count lessens in warmer environments, and given the close fit of tightie-whities, there is a correlation between low sperm count and tighter-fitting underwear. This is not the only medical explanation for low sperm count in men, but it may be a contributing factor.

CONDOMS. The variety of condoms on the market is boundless. An important factor you should keep in mind when choosing: lambskin condoms do not prevent STDs. Latex condoms are a must for protection and prevention.
PUTTING IT ON:
1. Buy condoms made of latex.
2. Whatever brand you prefer, invest in about a dozen of them and a cucumber. (Better yet, a pickle—you don't want to be making any unfavorable man/vegetable comparisons). First, practice opening up the package in one swift motion; if you consistently find this awkward, keep a small pair of scissors handy by the bed.
3. Next, inspect the condom carefully to see which direction it rolls over the head of the penis (or, in this case, the pickle). While rolling, always leave a little space at the top of the condom to catch the ejaculate. Practice this rolling-down motion with your eyes closed. Ideally, in the bedroom, you will be able to kiss your lover—thus distracting him a bit while rolling the condom down over the penis with one or both hands.
4. During withdrawal, hold the base of the condom to prevent semen from spilling. Do not try to use a condom more than once.
5. There are some women who are able to place the condom on the head of the penis, and then roll it down with their lips and tongue. Some consider this erotic; we consider it a circus trick. But if you think your lover might enjoy this, and you can do it without bursting out laughing, go right ahead.

Vagina

DISCHARGE. Every normal reproductive-aged woman produces discharge which changes in consistency and color throughout her monthly menstrual cycle. In the beginning of the month, discharge will appear scant and whitish.

During ovulation, in the middle of the month, it will become clear and thicker. Post-ovulation, at the end of the month, it will look whiter and stickier. If the discharge has a bad odor, itches, burns, becomes blood-tinged, or contains pus, then there is cause to be concerned and to see your gynecologist.

YEAST INFECTIONS. Yeast is a normal inhabitant of the vagina. When an overgrowth of yeast occurs, it will dominate the friendly yeast bacteria and kill it off, causing a thick, cottage-cheese-like discharge that is itchy and very uncomfortable. Yeast infections occur when there is excess heat and humidity inside the vagina, which spurs the overgrowth of the yeast inhabitant. Women using antibiotics are prone to getting yeast infections, because the antibiotic might kill off the friendly yeast. Diabetics are also prone to getting the infection. Of all vaginal infections, yeast infections are probably the most common, and are easily treatable by over-the-counter medications, available at pharmacies. If the problem persists for more than five days, you should consult your gynecologist.

DOUCHING. Commercial douches can affect the pH balance of the vagina, which can predispose you to infection and cause other problems. Keep it simple if you douche: water-and-baking-soda or water douches are the safest.

MORNING-AFTER CONTRACEPTION. The heat of the moment sweeps you off your feet, and leaves you frantic the next morning after the numbing realization of last night's negligence sets in. A condom breaking, missing a Pill, or just plain laziness can happen to the best of us. While there is no remedy for pre-period panic, there are forms of postcoital pregnancy intervention, none of which have been approved by the FDA. Consult a doctor for further information.
MORNING-AFTER SOLUTIONS THAT DON'T WORK:
1. Spermicide—doesn't work, unless you insert it one minute after ejaculation, and then it can get messy, and then you might be allergic to it. Enough said.

2. Douches—may even increase the likelihood of conception by pushing active sperm further up to the egg.

3. Hot baths—will make you feel relaxed and clean, but that's about it.

4. Chinese green tea—might calm your nerves, but a solution it is not.

MISSED PERIODS. If that little stick doesn't turn blue, there are many other reasons for missed menstrual cycles: a marked increase in exercise, for example, sudden and significant weight loss, or simple stress.

Sex

FANTASIES. Men and women fantasize about sex and erotic scenarios equally. Women who had sex 50 times or more a year had more sexual daydreams than women who had sex fewer than 50 times a year, according to a recent study. Frequent daydreamers also reported more closeness with their partners that was non-sexual. Both men and women need to be more tolerant of each other's fantasies. A fantasy is not an emotional longing; most of us are content to use fantasies to fuel the erotic imagination, rather than feeling compelled to act them out.

TOP FIVE FEMALE FANTASIES

1. *Making love with one's partner*
2. *Making love with a former lover or someone other than one's present partner*
3. *Sex in an erotic locale*
4. *Being forced to have sex against one's will with a trusted partner*
5. *Having sex in public while being watched*

"Having orgasms encourages the having of orgasms."

SUSIE BRIGHT

TOP FIVE MALE FANTASIES

1. *Being involved in a group*
2. *Watching others having sex*
3. *Making love in public*
4. *Having sex with a woman other than one's usual partner (a celebrity, neighbor, past lover, or friend)*
5. *Watching two women make love*

BIRTH CONTROL is everyone's personal decision. Safe sex is something else. The condom's original purpose—preventing conception—has now taken on new meaning—saving lives. Not practicing safe sex increases your chances of getting AIDS, which can kill you and others you love.

AIDS. The human immunodeficiency virus (HIV) causes the body to lose its immunity to disease. Once the virus infects the body, it replicates inside and subsequently destroys the white blood cells which help defend the body against a variety of infections and cancers. As the number of white blood cells decreases, the body becomes increasingly susceptible to opportunistic diseases. HIV lives in the blood and bodily fluids (semen and saliva). The main ways to transmit the virus are through sexual contact and sharing hypodermic needles. At the moment, there is no known cure for those infected with HIV, and no prospective cure. The best way to prevent transmission of HIV, besides abstinence, is the condom.

Buttocks

RASHES. These can occur on the buttocks when there is moisture buildup trapped between the skin and the underwear. Because buttocks spend most of their time covered by underwear, the skin's moisture doesn't get to air out, sometimes causing little red dots to form. Putting powder on the buttocks is helpful in preventing rashes. Staying in wet bathing suits can also spur rashes, so try to dry the buttocks area after getting it wet.

EXCESS HAIR. Hair on the buttocks is more acceptable for men than for women. It is normal in both sexes, but if you have darker hair and feel uncomfortable with it, you can wax or bleach excess hair.

"Sex is one of the most beautiful, wholesome, and natural things that money can buy."

STEVE MARTIN

HEMORRHOIDS are enlarged veins engorged with old and new blood that pop up through the skin near the rectum, appearing as hard, red bumps. They are caused by stress, constipation, high blood pressure, standing on your feet for prolonged periods of time, and overexertion. Extremely painful, hemorrhoids can afflict anyone at any age. Treatment includes over-the-counter lubricants that make the area around the rectum moist, allowing bowel movements to pass more easily, and provide a topical anesthetic to reduce pain. Pills are prescribed by a doctor in severe cases to soften the stool, making it easier to pass through the rectum. Sometimes an operation is necessary to remove the inflamed veins. If hemorrhoids do not go away within two weeks, and pain persists, see a doctor for further examination.

Hands

ARTHRITIS. Rheumatoid arthritis is a disease that attacks the joints by inflaming the joint muscles, making it difficult and painful to move. Because the hands have so many joints comprising and connecting each finger, they are a prime target for arthritis. Arthritis is a progressive disease which eventually destroys the joints and makes agility in motor-coordination tasks excruciatingly painful. Hard nodules form on the knuckles because of the buildup of joint swelling. Anti-inflammatory medication can be prescribed to quell pain, but no real cure has been found for this debilitating disease.

"Look at that! It's like . . . Jell-O on springs!"

JACK LEMMON

appreciating Marilyn Monroe's retreating derriere in Some Like It Hot

PREVENTING ARTHRITIS. About 16 million Americans suffer from osteoarthritis, the wearing down of joint cartilage. But even though some cartilage breakdown comes naturally with age, arthritis doesn't have to. The best methods of prevention are to lose excess weight (researchers think carrying excess baggage wears down the shock-absorbing capacity of the cartilage) and exercise—exercise keeps joints healthy—while avoiding injuries like torn knee ligaments and torn cartilage by preparing adequately and wearing the proper equipment.

CARPAL. Carpal tunnel syndrome, better known as the "typing disease," is the most commonly reported workplace injury. Continued wrist bending and pressure, which can be caused by excessive amounts of typing, leads to swelling of the tendons which pass through the narrow bony structure of the wrist wall, called the tunnel. As the tendons swell, they put pressure on the median nerve, which causes the pain. Treatment depends on how damaged the median nerve is. Operations are required in extreme cases; physical therapy suffices in less severe cases.
PREVENTION: When typing on computers, use curved keyboard wells—they are easier on the wrists—and wrist pads, which provide support by giving wrists leverage against the keyboard. Many keyboards can now be rotated to custom-fit the typist's hand.

CLAMMY HANDS. Clammy hands are, unfortunately, the barometer of our emotions: we only have to think about shaking hands with the boss, and our palms begin to drip.

There is no thoroughly satisfactory method for eradicating clamminess altogether, although frequent washing and avoiding caffeine when you're stepping into a tense situation have both been known to help.

KNUCKLE-CRACKING. Contrary to what your mother told you, there is no evidence that knuckle-cracking leads to arthritis later in life. (It's not even clear what makes that cracking sound, though it might be related to the snapping of gases in the joints.) But over many years, habitual cracking can lead to hand swelling, and some lessening of grip strength. So break the habit.

Nails

AVOIDING HANGNAILS. They're caused by dry skin. If you're prone to them, massage moisturizer onto your hands, being careful not to skip your cuticles and the base of your nails. Also, give yourself the occasional Vaseline treament: apply petroleum jelly to hands, and cover them with white cotton gloves while you sleep.

THE QUICK HOME MANICURE:
1. Soak in water for several minutes or apply moisturizer.
2. File nails both ways—with very tiny strokes—or else nail turns become tiny daggers. Don't file sides, where nail damage often starts. The shape you're aiming for is a round oval.
3. Don't use an orange stick to clean under nails; you might damage the skin underneath. Instead, soak them, and use a nailbrush to get rid of dirt.
4. The cuticle is meant to protect the nail by sealing off the opening between the nail and the skin. There's no need to cut the cuticles. Just moisturize them and push them back gently with fingertips or a towel.
5. Apply a base coat, polish, and top coat for shine. The key to a good manicure is the brush; you need a brush that's not so small it takes forever to spread the polish, and not so large the polish slops over the fingernail.

MALE NAILS. A well-manicured man's hand can be a beautiful thing, and for that all you need is an orangewood stick to scrape out dirt under nails and a clipper. (To use, clip with fingers turned toward your body for a square cut; otherwise your nails will have a tendency to lean, Pisa-like, in the direction you're trimming.)

"There are very simple ways to give a woman an orgasm. If you suspect that you don't know what you're doing but think you are bluffing effectively, and/or notice that it is taking more than a half hour, please be advised that you're fooling no one. It's just that most women are too polite or too concerned about the fragilities of the male ego to say anything. And, by the way, if you don't know what you're doing, for God's sake . . . DON'T DO IT HARDER!"

MERRILL MARKOE

Legs

SHIN SPLINTS. The name is deceiving because this injury—very common among runners—has nothing to do with the shins, but rather the muscles beneath them. Repeated impact on the shin muscles will make them splinter, causing considerable pain. The first rule is to stop exercising. Pain does not mean gain—throw Jane Fonda's words out the window! There's a difference between muscle ache from a good workout, and muscle pain. If any muscle is in pain stay off it. Apply ice and take Advil.

GROWING PAINS. Children may wake up in the middle of the night complaining that their legs ache. While there is no medical name for this condition, the best relief for leg cramps is a pain-relieving medication, and a good bedtime story.

SHAVING LEGS. **HOW TO:**
1. Allow hair to absorb water for about three minutes in the shower or bath. This will cause hairs to swell, and helps prevent skin irritation.
2. Use soap lather, shaving cream, or gel.
3. Use a sharp razor, and shave in the opposite direction from the direction in which the hairs grow, to get a smooth result.
4. Afterward, apply moisturizer to soothe skin and prevent those little razor bumps and rashes.

VARICOSE VEINS. **WHAT ARE THEY?** Either large, blue, and twisty, or small, pink, and spidery. When blood is heading downward through the arteries, it takes only the beating of the heart to speed it on its way. But on the way back up to the heart through the veins, blood flow is working against gravity. The vein system is supplied with one-way valves that snap shut behind the blood as it heads upstream. Sometimes the valves give out. Blood goes up, but also leaks backward through the valves. This blood then pools in the legs, and the result is swollen varicose veins.
AVOIDING THEM: For the most part, you can't; they're probably genetic—although

spending long parts of the day standing and constant crossing and uncrossing of legs both exacerbate the problem. Some patients have veins removed by laser or injected with a strong irritant; either way, the veins, no longer carrying blood, are not visible. More drastic treatment requires surgical "stripping" or removal of the vein, particularly if they're large, protruding, and ropy. (This is not as awful as it sounds. The veins next to the skin surface are doing only about 10 percent of the blood-pushing-up work; veins inside are doing the rest. So removing these surface veins doesn't seriously impede circulation.) While varicose veins can be uncomfortable, they're more of a cosmetic problem than a medical one, and they rarely demand treatment.

THIGH CREAM: **DOES IT WORK, AND IF IT DOES, WHY AREN'T YOU SLATHERED IN IT RIGHT NOW?**
The active ingredient in thigh cream is an asthma drug called aminophylline: when added to a cream and rubbed on thighs, it apparently reduces their circumference by as much as one inch. Researchers speculate the chemical works by dilating blood vessels and somehow helping to speed up fat metabolism in the area. Clinical trials haven't been completed. As with anything that sounds too good to be true, all we can do is hope.

Feet

Feet absorb the stress of our every step—two times our body weight, to be exact. By taking care of our feet, we can eliminate future problems that may occur if left unattended. Besides appearance-related problems, more serious conditions can arise, such as ankle, knee, and back pain, if we wear shoes that don't offer enough support. Fact: High heels can cause painful bunions and ankle problems. Tip: Shop for shoes in the late afternoon when feet are slightly swollen to avoid buying shoes too small. Opt for shoes with leather heels—they will conform best to your feet.

CALLUSES. These are layers of skin that build up over time due to shoes that are too tight or rub a part of the foot too much, causing extra layers of skin to form. The hard skin that forms serves to keep the skin from becoming raw and painful. The obvious prevention method is to wear shoes that fit. Keep the foot moist, either with petroleum jelly or body lotion. DON'T TRY TO FILE SKIN DOWN BY YOURSELF. If the callus doesn't go away by applying moisture, see a doctor.

CORNS AND BUNIONS. See a doctor to get them removed.

MASSAGE. A good foot massage can be a heavenly experience. Take the receiver's foot in your lap and press your fingertips all over the top of the foot (pressure depends on the receiver's preference). Then use thumbs to massage the outer edges of the sole in a circular pattern, pressing as you go. Do these motions slowly. Continue circling your thumbs inward until you reach the center of the sole. Body lotion or petroleum jelly is a good lubricant.

THE PEDICURE. Even a woman who would feel déclassée with a nail polish one shade bolder than palest pink can play the Dragon Lady with her toenail polish.
THE EASY PEDICURE:
1. Wash feet thoroughly in footbath until they're soft. Rub off callused skin with a pumice stone, soak again for a few minutes, and dry thoroughly with a towel.
2. Massage feet with a rich lotion.
3. Cut toenails straight across. Clean edges let air circulate beneath nails, preventing fungus and bacteria from growing.
4. Spread toes wide, either with cotton swabs or that cheap little gadget with the unfortunate name of "toe separator."
5. Apply the most vulgar nail polish you own. No one has to know. Wait for it to dry.
6. Smooth baby powder on feet. (For a male pedicure, follow steps 1, 2, 3, and 6, above. Forget 4 and 5, unless you're Ed Wood.)

Stress

PROBLEM-SOLVING TECHNIQUES. Classes in problem solving show the terminally stressed not only how to "fight down" whatever emotion they're feeling but also how to improve the situation that's causing it.

EXERCISE: Exercise may be the single most reliable form of relaxation—particularly for women, who, according to stress experts, have a higher

> "The abdomen is the reason why man does not easily take himself for a god."
>
> **FRIEDRICH NIETZSCHE**

rate of muscular problems from stress than men. Working up a sweat is extremely effective for flushing out toxins from the muscles and releasing tension. But forget about the "No pain, no gain" ethos of the '80s. When it starts to hurt, quit. Even if you cannot get to the gym or out to the tennis court during the day, you can do some physical movement to help release stress. For instance, gently teasing and relaxing muscles (starting at the toes and working upward) for 15 minutes a day will help relieve stress and improve concentration.

QUALITY TIME: Spend more time with friends and relatives. Families (well, some families) and friends can be great healers because they're our greatest source of loving bonds and connections. Our children, especially, allow us to shed our professional masks, and put us back in touch with our playfulness.

TASK MANAGEMENT: Manage tasks by breaking them down into smaller steps: make outlines, for example, or block out the day into hour or half-hour segments.

REWARDS: Create a system of rewards for yourself, rather than just punishments. A reward can be anything from a pampering manicure to a Caribbean vacation; the idea is to make room for more "downtime" in our days, and in our lives.

HOME SPA. HERBAL BATHS: Take a teaspoon each of rosemary, basil, dry mint, thyme, sage, and chamomile, tie them up in a cheesecloth bag, and suspend the bag under the bathtub while the water is running.

Sleep

TO AVOID SNORING. More than 300 anti-snoring devices are registered at the U.S. Patent Office, a reflection of our national desperation to cure the offending snorer. Usually a nudge will force the snorer to change position and cease his drone temporarily, but the only permanent solution is surgical: the procedure trims away excess tissue and removes the back half of the soft palate, which is then stretched taut. The result? No excess tissue when the throat relaxes—and an unimpaired breathing space.

Food

VITAMINS. The debate among nutritionists is whether we should all be taking vitamin supplements, or whether most of us get all the vitamins we need from our diets. Currently, 40 percent of American adults take them. Studies have shown people taking 300 to 500 milligrams of vitamin C had a 25 to 45 percent lower death rate from heart disease, and a 10 to 42 percent reduced mortality from all causes. There are also studies demonstrating that vitamin overdoses can be dangerous: A and D, fat-soluble vitamins that get stored in body tissues, can accumulate to toxic levels. It appears that a daily multivitamin, or daily doses of vitamins E, C, and beta-carotene, may be beneficial and at worst won't hurt.

> "I have gained and lost the same ten pounds so many times over and over again, my cellulite must have déjà vu."
>
> **JANE WAGNER**

where.

Taking care of your body means different things to different people. From a haircut to a physical, a massage to a workout—enjoying and appreciating your body can often be enhanced, sometimes by products and sometimes by instruction or guidance. The resources are endless but one always needs a place to start.

UNITED STATES

ARIZONA

SPA

ARLINGTON HOTEL
Central Avenue at Fountain Street
Hot Springs, AZ 71902
800/643-1502
(Old hot-springs resort)

CANYON RANCH
8600 East Rockcliff Road
Tucson, AZ 85715
800/726-9900
(Ultramodern fitness spa)

ELIZABETH ARDEN'S MAINE CHANCE
5830 East Jean Avenue
Phoenix, AZ 85018
602/947-6365
(Relaxation spa)

THE PHOENICIAN
6000 East Camelback Road
Scottsdale, AZ 85251
800/888-8234
(Upscale resort hotel and spa)

CALIFORNIA

COSMETICS

BARE ESSENTIALS
Three Embarcadero Center
San Francisco, CA 94111
415/391-2830
(Bath and body products)

GEORGETTE KLINGER SALON
312 North Rodeo Drive
Beverly Hills, CA 90210
310/274-6347
(Hair removal)

KATE ELLIOT BEAUTY BASICS
19826 Ventura Boulevard
Woodland Hills, CA 91364
818/883-4445
(Aromatherapy, soaps, gels, oils)

OCEANS OF LOTIONS
842 Cole Street
San Francisco, CA 94117
415/566-2326
(Bath, body, natural cosmetics)

SKIN ZONE
575 Castro Street
San Francisco, CA 94114
415/626-7933
(Body, skin, hair-care products)

VOTRE BEAUTÉ SKIN CARE SALON
3263 Sacramento Street
San Francisco, CA 94115
415/563-2420
(Hair removal)

MEDICINAL

BEAUTY KLINIEK AROMATHERAPY DAY SPA
3268 Governor Drive
San Diego, CA 92122
619/457-0191
(Manicures with essential oils)

CRISTINA FIORE ITALIAN SKIN CARE SALON
1150 Coast Village Road
Santa Barbara, CA 93108
800/826-1392
(Skin-care salon)

GEORGE MICHAEL OF MADISON AVENUE
9885 Little Santa Monica Boulevard
Beverly Hills, CA 90210
310/282-0957
(Hair salon specializing in long hair)

HOMEOPATHIC COMPANY
629 Broadway
Santa Monica, CA 90401
310/395-1131
(Major homeopathic remedies)

IN HARMONY HERBS AND SPICES
4808 Santa Monica Avenue
San Diego, CA 92107
619/223-8051
(Organic and wild-crafted herbs)

JET.RHYS SALON
3846 Fifth Avenue
San Diego, CA 92103
619/291-7511
(Long, natural styles; coloring)

JOSÉ EBER SALON
224 North Rodeo Drive
Beverly Hills, CA 90210
310/278-7646
(Cutting-edge fashion cuts)

LINDA KAMMINS AROMATHERAPY SALON
848 North La Cienega Boulevard,
Suite 2104
Los Angeles, CA 90069
310/659-6257
(Restore hair to natural balance with herb and vegetable aromatherapy)

LOUIS LICARI COLOR GROUP
450 North Canon Drive
Beverly Hills, CA 90210
310/247-0855;
also in NYC, original salon,
212/517-8084

HAHNEMANN MEDICAL CLINIC
PHARMACY, INC.
828 San Pablo Avenue
Albany, CA 94706
510/527-3003
(Major homeopathic remedies)

JESSICA NAIL CLINIC
8627 Sunset Boulevard
Los Angeles, CA 90069
310/659-9292
(Customized treatments)

MICHAELJOHN
414 North Camden Drive
Beverly Hills, CA 90210
310/278-8333
(Facials, manicures, body waxing)

PENNINGTON SALON
139 South Kings Road
Los Angeles, CA 90048
213/653-4981
(African-American hair specialist)

STEPHEN SAIZ SALON
275 Post Street
San Francisco, CA 94108
415/398-2345
(The latest hip looks)

TABOO
8446 West 3rd Street
Los Angeles, CA 90048
213/655-3770
(Temporary color processes)

VISIONS
8019 Melrose Avenue
Los Angeles, CA 90046
213/651-4545
(Mostly subtle coloring)

SPA

BEAUTY BODY WELLNESS
2325 Third Street, Suite 321
San Francisco, CA 94107
415/626-4685
(Full-service holistic day spa/salon)
Catalogue / Mail Order

BEVERLY HOT SPRINGS
308 North Oxford Avenue
Los Angeles, CA 90004
213/734-7000
(Day spa)

ESALEN INSTITUTE
Big Sur, CA 93920
408/667-3000
(Natural hot springs)

GOLDEN DOOR
777 Deer Springs Road
San Marcos, CA 92069
800/424-0777
(Deluxe spa and resort for women)

IL MAKIAGE
323 Geary Street, Suite 606
San Francisco, CA 94102
800/685-4673
(Full-service day spa and salon)

LA COSTA RESORT & SPA
2100 Costa Del Mar Road
Carlsbad, CA 92009
619/438-9111
(Fitness, aromatherapy, massages)

MAURO
8306 Melrose Avenue
Los Angeles, CA 90069
213/653-4530
(Natural hair treatments)

PRESTON WYNNE SPA
14567 Big Basin Way
Saratoga, CA 95070
408/741-5525
(Holistic day spa)

SONOMA MISSION INN & SPA
P.O. Box 1447
Sonoma, CA 95476
800/862-4945 in Calif.; 800/358-9022
(Spa/resort in wine country)

THE SPA
AT L'AUBERGE DEL MAR
1540 Camino Del Mar
Del Mar, CA 92014
619/259-1515
(Seaside spa)

THE SPA HOTEL AND MINERAL
SPRINGS
100 North Indian Canyon Drive
Palm Springs, CA 92262
619/325-1461
(Mineral baths)

TWO BUNCH PALMS
RESORT & SPA
67-425 Two Bunch Palms Trail
Desert Hot Springs, CA 92240
619/329-8791 or 800/472-4334
(Casual and private desert spa)

VERA'S RETREAT IN THE GLEN
2980 Beverly Glen Circle
Suite 100
Los Angeles, CA 90077
310/470-6362
(Day spa)

COLORADO

COSMETICS

ALFALFA'S MARKET
1651 Broadway
Boulder, CO 80302
303/442-0909 for statewide listings
(Fresh and dry botanicals, all-natural)

MEDICINAL

WISHGARDEN HERBS
1308 Kilkenny Street
Boulder, CO 80303
303/665-9508
(Herbalist, childbearing preparations)

SALON

INTERHAIR
3150 East Third Avenue
Denver, CO 80206
303/377-3377
(Soft, natural styles)

SPA

PEAKS AT TELLURIDE
136 Country Club Drive
Telluride, CO 81435
800/789-2220 or 303/728-6800
(Full-service spa, winter skiing)

OXFORD AVEDA SPA & SALON
1616 Seventeenth Street
Denver, CO 80202
303/628-5435
(Day spa, full-service health club)

CONNECTICUT

COSMETICS

DECLEOR USA, INC.
500 West Avenue
Stamford, CT 06902
800/722-2219
(French aromatherapy, skin-care line)

SPA

NORWICH INN AND SPA
607 West Thames Street
Norwich, CT 06360
203/886-2401
(Progressive relaxation spa)

FLORIDA

MEDICINAL

BUDGET PHARMACY
3001 NW 7th Street
Miami, FL 33125
800/221-9772
(Major homeopathic remedies)

SALON

SKIN APEEL DAY SPA
21301 Powerline Road, Suite 215
Boca Raton, FL 33433
407/852-8081
(Botanical manicures)

SPA

DORAL SATURNIA
INTERNATIONAL SPA RESORT
8755 NW 36th Street
Miami, FL 33178
800/331-7768
(Full-service spa/resort)

**SAFETY HARBOR SPA &
FITNESS CENTER**
105 North Bayshore Drive
Safety Harbor, FL 34695
800/237-0155
(Natural mineral springs resort)

**THE PALM-AIRE SPA &
RESORT**
2601 Palm-Aire Drive North
Pompano Beach, FL 33069
305/972-3300 or 800/272-5624
(Various massage techniques)

WILLIAMS ISLAND SPA
5300 Island Boulevard
Williams Island, FL 33160
305/937-7860
(Day spa)

GEORGIA

SALON

SCOTT COLE SALON
2859 Piedmont Road NE
Atlanta, GA 30305
404/237-4970
(Coloring and highlights)

VAN MICHAEL'S
39 West Paces Ferry Road
Atlanta, GA 30350
404/237-4664
(Contemporary, low-maintenance cuts)

SPA

NATURAL BODY DAY SPA
273 East Paces Ferry Road NE
Atlanta, GA 30305
404/841-9554
(Herbal day spa, mud baths)

ILLINOIS

MEDICINAL

MERZ APOTHECARY
4716 North Lincoln Avenue
Chicago, IL 60625
312/989-0900
(Homeopathic remedies)

SALON

ART + SCIENCE
811 Church Street
Evanston, IL 60201
708/864-HAIR
(Classic, tailored cuts)

MARCO BONNÉ
701 North Michigan Avenue
Chicago, IL 60611
312/321-0295
(Coloring)

TRIO SALON
11 East Walton Street
Chicago, IL 60611
312/944-6999
(Easy-care cuts, colorists)

SPA

**MARIO TRICOCI HAIR SALON
AND DAY SPA**
277 East Ontario Street
Chicago, IL 60611
312/915-0960
(Day spa)

THE HEARTLAND SPA
R.R. 1, Box 181
Gilman, IL 60938
815/683-2182 or 800/545-4893
(Lakefront spa/resort)

MASSACHUSETTS

MEDICINAL

**NORTHEAST HOMEOPATHIC
PRODUCTS DIVISION OF
ACTON PHARMACY**
563 Massachusetts Avenue
Acton, MA 01720
800/551-3611
(Homeopathic remedies)
Catalogue / Mail Order

SALON

BOTANICAL REX
39 Newbury Street
Boston, MA 02116
617/859-5959
(Day spa, eco-sensitive skin care)

MARIO RUSSO
9 Newbury Street
Boston, MA 02116
617/424-6676
(Hair treatments and massage)

SAFAR COIFFURE
235 Newbury Street
Boston, MA 02116
617/247-3933
(Natural hair treatments)

SPA

**CANYON RANCH IN THE
BERKSHIRES**
165 Kemble Street
Lenox, MA 01240
800/726-9900
(Baths and massage, fitness spa)

THE DAY SPA
1640 Massachusetts Avenue
Lexington, MA 02173
617/861-7722
(Day spa)

NEW MEXICO

SPA

TEN THOUSAND WAVES
Hyde Park Road
Santa Fe, NM 87504
505/982-9304
(Japanese health spa)

NEW YORK

SPA

CRYSTAL SPA
92 South Broadway
Saratoga Springs, NY 12866
518/584-2556
(Spa)

**GURNEY'S INN RESORT
AND SPA**
Old Montauk Highway
Montauk, NY 11954
516/668-2509
(Baths and massage)

THE SAGAMORE RESORT
110 Sagamore Road
Bolton Landing, NY 12814
800/358-3585
(Baths and massage)

NEW YORK CITY

COSMETICS

AD HOC SOFTWARES
410 West Broadway
New York, NY 10012
212/925-2652
(Bath/body lotions and accessories)

ADAH LEZORGEN
Pierre Michel Salon, Plaza Hotel
Fifth Avenue at Central Park South
New York, NY 10019
212/593-7930
(Makeup artist, lessons)

ARSI, LTD. SKIN CARE CLINIC
162 West 56th Street, Suite 206
New York, NY 10019
212/582-5720
(Hair removal, herbal wax)

BATH & BODY WORKS
89 South Street, Pier 17
New York, NY 10038
212/693-0247
(Bath oils, soaps, body lotions)

BATH ISLAND
469 Amsterdam Avenue
New York, NY 10024
212/787-9415
(Bath products)

BERGDORF GOODMAN
754 Fifth Avenue
New York, NY 10019
212/753-7300
(Bath and skin products)

BLOOMINGDALE'S
59th Street at Lexington Avenue
New York, NY 10022
212/355-5900 for U.S. listings
(Bath and skin products)

BOBBI BROWN
Frederic Fekkai Beauty Center
Bergdorf Goodman
1 West 57th Street
New York, NY 10019
212/753-9500
(Makeup artist, lessons)

CHANEL BOUTIQUE
5 East 57th Street
New York, NY 10022
212/355-5050
(Cosmetics)

CRABTREE & EVELYN
520 Madison Avenue
New York, NY 10022
212/758-6419
(Bath and body products)

DONNA KARAN BEAUTY COMPANY
550 Seventh Avenue
New York, NY 10018
800/647-7474
(Bath and body products)

ELIZABETH ARDEN
691 Fifth Avenue
New York, NY 10022
212/546-0200
(Salon)

EMPORIO ARMANI
110 Fifth Avenue
New York, NY 10011
212/727-3240; or 212/570-1122 for international listings
(Soaps and bath oils)

ERBE
196 Spring Street
New York, NY 10012
212/966-1445
(Herbal beauty center)

FELISSIMO
10 West 56th Street
New York, NY 10022
212/956-4438
(Bath and skin products)

FREDERIC FEKKAI BEAUTY CENTER
Bergdorf Goodman
1 West 57th Street
New York, NY 10019
212/753-9500
(Full-service salon)

GOODEBODIES
330 Columbus Avenue
New York, NY 10023
212/721-9317
(Loofahs, bath oils, gels)
Catalogue / Mail Order

H₂O
650 Madison Avenue
New York, NY 10022
212/767-5986; or 800/242-BATH for listings in the U.S. and Canada
(Bath, beauty, aromatherapy)

JOHN ALLEN MEN'S SALON
95 Trinity Place
New York, NY 10006
212/406-3000
(Barbershop)

KIEHL'S
109 Third Avenue
New York, NY 10003
212/475-3400
(Bath and skin products)

PHYTOTHÉRATHRIE
625 Madison Avenue
New York, NY 10022
212/754-2300
(French botanical hair-product line)

SALON ISHI
70 East 55th Street
New York, NY 10022
212/888-ISHI
(Japanese herbal salon, hair removal)

TAKASHIMAYA
693 Fifth Avenue
New York, NY 10022
212/350-0100
(Skin-care and bath products)

ZONA
97 Greene Street
New York, NY 10012
212/925-6750
(Bath and body products)

MEDICINAL

ANGELICA'S TRADITIONAL HERBS AND SPICES
147 First Avenue
New York, NY 10003
212/529-4335
(Collection of Western/Chinese herbs)

BIGELOW CHEMISTS
414 Avenue of the Americas
New York, NY 10011
212/533-2700
(Major homeopathic remedies)
Catalogue / Mail Order

SALON

ARTÉ SALON
284 Lafayette Street
New York, NY 10012
212/941-5932
(Cuts and treatment)

BENDEL'S
712 Fifth Avenue
New York, NY 10019
212/247-1100
(Cuts and treatment)

COPPOLA
673 Madison Avenue
New York, NY 10021
212/752-7770
(Hair salon)

HAIME MUÑOZ
882 Lexington Avenue, Studio 3
New York, NY 10021
212/861-3414
(Hair straightening)

HELEN LEE DAY SPA
205 East 60th Street
New York, NY 10022
800/288-1077
(Chinese herbal salon)

J. F. LAZARTIGUE
764 Madison Avenue
New York, NY 10021
212/288-2250
(Hair products)

JACQUES DESSANGE
505 Park Avenue
New York, NY 10022
212/308-1400
(Hair products and treatment)

LUIS GUY D
41 East 57th Street
New York, NY 10022
212/753-6077
(Natural-looking color)

MINARDI SALON
29 East 61st Street
New York, NY 10021
212/308-1711
(Colorist and consultant for Clairol)

THE ORIBE SALON
691 Fifth Avenue
New York, NY 10022
212/319-3910
(Hip and conservative coloring)

SALON DADA
4 West 16th Street
New York , NY 10011
212/741-DADA
(Hair treatment and scalp treatment)

SPA

CATHERINE ATZEN DAY SPA
856 Lexington Avenue
New York, NY 10021
212/517-2400
(Day spa)

THE GREAT AMERICAN BACKRUB
958 Third Avenue
New York, NY 10022
212/832-1766
(The 8½-minute massage, $8)

MILLEFLEURS
13-17 Laight Street
New York, NY 10013
212/966-3656
(Eclectic day spa)

RUSSIAN BATHS
268 East 10th Street
New York, NY 10009
212/674-9250
(Russian/Turkish baths, massage)

OREGON

MEDICINAL

**WILDFLOWERS ON
HAWTHORNE**
3202 SE Hawthorne Boulevard
Portland, OR 97214
503/230-9485
(Organic and wild-crafted herbs)

SALON

JACKIE CROMER'S BOB SHOP
555 Southwest Oak Street
Portland, OR 97204
503/226-2886
(Hair care and corrective coloring)

TEXAS

MEDICINAL

**ACUPUNCTURE AND
AESTHETICS CENTER**
17194 Preston Road, Suite 222
Dallas, TX 75248
214/380-9070
(Treats skin problems)

SALON

JACQUES DESSANGE
1800 Post Oak Boulevard, Suite 192,
Saks Pavilion
Houston, TX 77056
713/960-1010
(Fits cuts to your lifestyle)

PAUL NEINAST SALON
4524 Cole Avenue
Dallas, TX 75205
214/521-4300
(Coloring)

SPA

THE GREENHOUSE
P.O. Box 1144
Arlington , TX 76004-1144
817/640-4000
(Elegant spa/resort for women)

NEPENTHE DAY SPA
3519 Cedar Springs Road
Dallas, TX 75219
214/521-3311
(Day spa)

THE PHOENIX SPA
111 North Post Oak Lane
Houston, TX 77024
713/685-6836
(Exercise, diet, stress management)

VERMONT

SPA

THE EQUINOX
Historic Route 7A
Manchester Village, VT 05254
802/362-4700 or 800/362-4747
(Baths and massage)

THE SPA AT TOPNOTCH
4000 Mountain Road
Stowe, VT 05672
802/253-6463 or 800/451-8686
(Baths and massage)

WASHINGTON

SALON

GARY BOCZ
1523 Sixth Avenue
Seattle, WA 98101
206/624-9134
(Individualized color treatments)

OBADIAH
2123A First Avenue
Seattle, WA 98121
206/448-7820
(Outrageous color treatments)

SPA

**ILDIKO'S SKIN AND BODY
SALON**
705 Broadway East
Seattle, WA 98102
206/328-4311
(Elegant day spa)

WEST VIRGINIA

SPA

THE GREENBRIER
West Main Street
White Sulphur Springs, WV 24986
304/536-1110
(Natural sulfur springs baths)

NATIONAL LISTINGS

COSMETICS

THE BODY SHOP
45 Horsehill Road
Cedar Knolls, NJ 07927
201/984-9200 for U.S. listings; or
71/436-5681 for U.K. listings
(Bath and body products)

NEIMAN MARCUS
1618 Main Street
Dallas, TX 75201
214/741-6911
(Bath and skin-care products)

ORIGINS
402 West Broadway
New York, NY 10012
212/219-9764; or
800/723-7310 for U.S. listings
(Bath and skin-care products)

PARISIAN
2100 River Chase Galleria
Birmingham, AL 35244
205/987-4200; or
205/940-4000 for U.S. listings
(Cosmetics and skin-care products)

RICH'S
Lenox Square Shopping Mall
3393 Peachtree Road
Atlanta, GA 30326
404/231-2611
(Fine bath products)

MEDICINAL

DOLISOS AMERICA, INC.
3014 Rigel Avenue
Las Vegas, NV 89102
800/365-4767
(Major homeopathic remedies)

PENN HERB COMPANY
603 North Second Street
Philadelphia, PA 19123
215/925-3336
(Large selection of dried herbs)

MAIL ORDER

COSMETICS

AROMA VERA
5901 Rodeo Road
Los Angeles, CA 90016
800/669-9514
(Special blends for body and bath)

AVON
800/FOR-AVON
(Personal bath products)

BURT'S BEES
308 West Hillsboro Street
Creedmore, NC 27522
919/528-0064
(Beeswax-based products)

ECCO BELLA
125 Pompton Plains Crossroad
Wayne, NJ 07470
201/616-0220
(Cruelty-free body products)

GOODEBODIES
330 Columbus Avenue
New York, NY 10023
212/721-9317
(Loofahs, bath oils, gels)

**PENHALIGON'S PERFUMERS
LTD.**
41 Wellington Street
London WC2E 7BN
UK
71/836-2150; or
81/880-2050 for mail order
(Old-fashioned English scents)

REAL GOODS TRADING CORP.
966 Mazzoni Street
Ukiah, CA 95482
800/762-7325
(Eco body and hair-care products)

SIMPLERS BOTANICAL CO.
P.O. Box 39
Forestville, CA 95436
707/887-2012
(Natural body/bath oils and creams)

MEDICINAL

BIGELOW CHEMISTS
414 Avenue of the Americas
New York, NY 10011
212/533-2700
(Major homeopathic remedies)

BOERICKE & TAFEL
800/876-9505
(Homeopathic products by mail)

BOIRON
800/BLU-TUBE
(Homeopathic products by mail)

BUDGET PHARMACY
3001 NW 7th Street
Miami, FL 33125
800/221-9772
(Major homeopathic remedies)

HERB PRODUCTS
11012 Magnolia Boulevard
North Hollywood, CA 91691
213/877-3104
(Domestic and imported herbs)

THE HERBALIST
6500 20th Avenue NE
Seattle, WA 98115
206/523-2600
(Large selection of dried herbs)

HERBS, ETC.
323 Aztec Street
Santa Fe, NM 87501
505/471-6488
(Huge selection of herbs for brewing,
cooking, and medicinal use)

JONES DRUG COMPANY
1060 North Campbell Avenue
Tucson, AZ 85719
602/881-1228
(Major homeopathic remedies)

PENN HERB COMPANY
603 North Second Street
Philadelphia, PA 19123
215/925-3336
(Large selection of dried herbs)

**STANDARD HOMEOPATHIC
COMPANY**
800/624-9659
(Homeopathic products by mail)

WINTER SUN TRADING CO.
107 North San Francisco Street, Suite 1
Flagstaff, AZ 86001
602/774-2884
(Organic and wild-crafted herbs)

TOYS

GOOD VIBRATIONS
1210 Valencia at 23rd Street
San Francisco, CA 94110
415/974-8990
(Sex toys, books, and movies)

INTERNATIONAL
LISTINGS

CANADA

BRITISH COLUMBIA

SPA

**HARRISON HOT SPRINGS
VILLA HOTEL**
P.O. Box 389, 270 Esplanade
British Columbia V0M 1K0
604/796-9339
(Natural hot springs)

MONTREAL

COSMETICS

EATON
677 rue Sainte-Catherine Ouest
514/284-8484
(Skin care and body care)

FRANCE

SPA

ATLANTHAL
153 boulevard des Plages
Anglet-Chiberta
64600
59/52-75-75
(Atlantic coast spa town)

HOTEL HERMITAGE
Esplanade François-André
La Baule 44504
40/11-46-36
(A stylish spa on the Atlantic coast)

HOTEL NORMANDY
38 rue Jean-Mermoz
Deauville
14800
31/98-66-22
(Thalassotherapy treatments)

HOTEL ROYAL
Rive Sud du Lac de Genève
Évian-les-Bains
74500
50/26-85-00
(Elegant spa town)

**INSTITUT DE
THALASSOTHÉRAPIE**
11 rue Louison-Bobet
Biarritz
64200
59/24-20-80
(Baths, injuries treatment, massage)

LES PRÉS D'EUGÉNIE
Thermes d'Eugénie
Eugénie-les-Bains
40320
58/05-06-06
(Baths, nouvelle cuisine, medical
treatments, massage)

**TRIANON PALACE AND
TRIANON PALACE HOTEL**
1 boulevard de la Reine
Versailles
78000
30/84-38-00
(Spa, cellulite treatments)

PARIS

COSMETICS

ANNE PARÉE
10 rue Duphot
75001
42/60-52-82
(Beauty store)

ANNICK GOUTAL
14 rue de Castiglione
75001
45/51-36-13 for Paris listings
(Perfume, soaps, body lotions)

BEAUTÉ DIVINE
40 rue Saint-Sulpice
75006
43/26-25-31
(Bathroom accessories)

DIPTYQUE
34 boulevard Saint-Germain
75005
43/26-45-27
(Known for its soaps and toiletries)

GUERLAIN
68 avenue des Champs-Élysées
75008
47/89-71-00
(Perfumes and toilet waters)

**HERBORISTERIE PALAIS
ROYAL**
11 rue des Petits Champs
75001
42/97-54-68
(Body lotions and shampoos)

L'ARTISAN PARFUMEUR
24 boulevard Raspail
75007
42/22-23-32
(Beauty store)

P. DE NICOLAI
69 avenue Raymond-Poincaré
75016
47/55-90-44
(Beauty store)

PAIN D'ÉPICE
35 passage Jouffroy
75016
47/55-90-44
(Beauty store)

PHARMACIE LECLERC
10 rue Vignon
75009
47/42-04-59
(Beauty store)

SAPONIFÈRE
Forum des Halles
75001
40/39-92-14
(Beauty store)

SEPHORA
50 rue de Passy
75016
45/20-03-15
(Cosmetics supermarket)

MEDICINAL

LA PHARMACIE PIQUET
18 rue Jean-Nicot
75007
47/05-17-88
(Homeopathic preparations)

GERMANY

SPA

BRENNER'S PARK HOTEL
Schillerstrasse 426
Baden Baden
76530
7/221-9000
(Spa, medical treatments)

GREAT BRITAIN
COSMETICS

COSMETICS TO GO
Freepost, Poole
Dorset
BH15 1BR
800/373-366
(Personal bath products)
Catalogue / Mail Order

CONDOMANIA
Unit 5, Rivermead
Piper's Way
Thatcham
RG13 4EP
63/587-4393
(Personal bath products)
Catalogue / Mail Order

LONDON

COSMETICS

CULPEPER THE HERBALISTS
21 Bruton Street
Berkeley Square
London W1X 7DA
71/629-4559
(Herbs, spices, cosmetics)

THE BEAUTY CLINIC
413A Fulham Palace Road
SW6
71/736-7676
(Beauty products)

THE BODY SHOP
137 Kensington High Street
W8
71/376-0771; call for national listings
(Natural skin-care products)

D. R. HARRIS & CO. LTD.
29 St. James's Street
SW1A
71/930-3915
(Men's skin-care products)

FLORIS
89 Jermyn Street
W1Y 6JH
71/930-2885
(Fragrances, oils, soaps, lotions)

GEORGE F. TRUMPER
9 Curzon Street
W1Y 7FL
71/499-1850
(Men's toiletries)

HACKETT
136-138 Sloane Street
W1
71/730-3331
(Men's toiletries)

**JAMES BODENHAM &
COMPANY**
88 Jermyn Street
SW1Y
71/930-5340
(Bath oils and gels, lotions)

**MOLTON BROWN
HAIRDRESSING**
58 South Molton Street
W1
71/629-1872
(Body and hair products)

THE NAIL PLACE
231 Oxford Street
W1
71/439-0451
(Manicures)

PENHALIGON'S
16 Burlington Arcade
Piccadilly W1
71/629-1416
(Body products for men and women)

SELFRIDGES, LTD.
Oxford Street
W1A 1AB
71/629-1234
(Bath products, furnishings)

MEDICINAL

**BEAUCHAMP FOOT & BODY
CARE**
48 Beauchamp Place
SW3 1NX
71/225-0794

HOLLAND & BARRETT
Unit C12, West 1 Shopping Centre
Bond Street Station
W1
71/493-7988
(Health products)

NEALS YARD REMEDIES
15 Neals Yard
14 Covent Garden
WC2
71/379-7222
(Body products and cosmetics)

THE SANCTUARY
12 Floral Street
WC2 E9DH
71/240-9635
(Health products)

SALON

HARRODS: HAIR & BEAUTY
Knightsbridge
SW1
71/581-2021
(Hair and makeup)

HARVEY NICHOLS
109 Knightsbridge
SW1
71/235-7208
(Hair and makeup)

VIDAL SASSOON
60 South Molton Street
W1Y
71/491-8848 for national listings
(Hair)

SPA

CHAMPNEYS HEALTH RESORT
Champneys at Tring
Hertfordshire
HP23 6HY
442/873-155
(Luxury spa)

**GRAYSHOTT HALL & LEISURE
CENTRE**
Grayshott, near Hindhead
Surrey GU26 6JJ
428/604-331
(Health/fitness spa)

LUCKNAM PARK
Colerne
Wiltshire SN14 8AZ
225/74-27-77
(Georgian country-house spa)

**SHRUBLAND HALL HEALTH
CLINIC**
Coddenham, near Ipswich
Suffolk IP6 9QH
473/83-04-04
(A palatial Georgian manor house)

LONDON

THE DORCHESTER SPA
The Dorchester
Park Lane W1A 2HJ
71/629-8888
(Spa)

.PORCHESTER SPA
Porchester Road
Queensway
W2
71/792-3980
(Public baths)

ITALY

SPA

GRAND HOTEL E LA PACE
Viale Della Torretta
Montecatini Terme 51016
5/72-75801
(Italy's most elegant spa town)

**GRAND HOTEL PUNTA
MOLINO**
Lungomare Cristoforo Colombo
Ischia Porto I-80077
81/99-15-44
(Thermal springs)

HOTEL CASTEL RUNDEG
Via Scena 2
Merano 39012
473-34100
(Hot springs resort)

TERME DI MONTECANTI
Viale Verdi 41
Montecatini Terme 51016
39/572-7781
(Spa, mud baths)

TERME DI SATURNIA HOTEL
Saturnia (Grosetto) 58050
564/601-061
(Spa)

TERME REGINA ISABELLA
Piazza St. Restituta
Lacco Ameno 80076
Ischia
81/99-43-22
(Baths, volcanic muds, massage)

MILAN

COSMETICS

VECCHIA
Via San Giovanni Sul Muro 8
391/87-36-51
(Milan's most elegant profumeria)

SALON

**MARIA BRUNA BEAUTY
WORKSHOP**
Piazza Vescovato 1C
Brescia (near Milan)
3/04-51-94

ROME

SALON

**FEMME SISTINA BEAUTY
CENTER**
Via Sistina 75A
6/678-0260

JAPAN

TOKYO

COSMETICS

MITSUKOSHI
1-4-1 Nihonbashi
Muromachi Chuo-ku
3/3241-3311
(Skin-care and bath products)

PARCO
14 Udagawa-cho
Shibuya-ku
3/3464-5111
(Skin-care and bath products)

SPIRAL MARKET
Spiral Bldg. 2F, 5-6-23
Minami Aoyama, Minato-ku
3/3498-5792
(Herbs)

TAKASHIMAYA
2-4-1 Nihonbashi
Chuo-ku
3/3211-4111
(Skin-care and bath products)

TINA MARRY
20-13 Sarugaku-cho
Shibuya-ku
3/5489-9800 or 3/5489-5111
(Scented skin-care and bath products)

SALON

MOD'S HAIR
Twin Minami Aoyama Bldg. 1F
3-14-13 Minami Aoyama, Minato-ku
3/3478-0131
(Hair salons)

RESOURCES

cover **SHELLS** - courtesy of Kenji Toma

12–13 **SHELLS** - courtesy of Kenji Toma

26 **GEARS** - courtesy of Mark Weiss

28 **LOTUS LEAF** - courtesy of Ted Muehling

38–39 **BLUE BONE** - Evolution, NYC

40 **AMMONITE** - Evolution, NYC

52 **VINTAGE HAND MIRRORS** - courtesy of Ted Muehling

84–85 **ALUMINUM COMB** - Ray's Beauty Supply; **TORTOISESHELL COMB** - Hackett, London

89 **CURLERS** - Ray's Beauty Supply

91 **HAIRCUTTING SHEARS** - Hackett, London

92 **HAIRBRUSH** - Aveda Esthetique

105 **ASSORTMENT OF SPONGES AND PUMICE STONES** - Felissimo

109 **FRAGRANCE BOTTLES:** small blue bottle - Felissmo; large blue bottle - Barneys; others - Brosse, USA, Inc.

118 **UNDERWEAR** - Dolce & Gabbana

130 **CLEAVER** - courtesy of Dean & Deluca

140 **KEYHOLE** - Urban Archaeology

152 **MEXICAN CROSS OF LIMBS** - courtesy of Robert Valentine

168 **SCALE** - Eclectic Encore

182 **BOOT** - courtesy of Jeff Stone

190 **SKULL** - Evolution

QUOTES

2 Oscar Wilde, *The Picture of Dorian Gray*, 1891

6 Australian Aboriginal saying

16 Gloria Steinem, *Revolution from Within* (Little, Brown and Company, 1992)

19 William Shakespeare, *Hamlet*

21 Deepak Chopra, *Ageless Body, Timeless Mind* (Harmony Books, 1993)

23 Naomi Wolf, *The Beauty Myth* (Morrow, 1991)

30–31 Dean Ornish, *Reversing Heart Disease* (Random House, 1990)

32 Oscar Wilde, *The Picture of Dorian Gray*, 1891

46 Oscar Wilde, *The Picture of Dorian Gray*, 1891

53 Dorothy Parker, *The Penguin Book of Modern Humorous Quotations* (Penguin Books, 1987)

54 Naomi Wolf, *The Beauty Myth* (Morrow, 1991)

72 Howard Hughes, *The Penguin Book of Modern Humorous Quotations* (Penguin Books, 1987)

77 Ogden Nash, *Just Joking*, portions by Donald L. Smith, portions by Jon Winokur (WordStar International, 1992)

87 Hubert de Givenchy, *Vogue*, July 1985

91 Julio Cortázar, *The Winners*

94–95 Fran Lebowitz, *Just Joking*, portions by Donald L. Smith, portions by Jon Winokur (WordStar International, 1992)

98 Tom Lehrer, *National Brotherhood Week*

104 Martha Graham, *The New York Times*, March 31, 1985

112 P. G. Wodehouse, *The Penguin Dictionary of Modern Humorous Quotations* (Penguin Books, 1987)

122–23 Gloria Steinem, *Revolution from Within* (Little, Brown and Company, 1992)

124 Colette, *Gigi*

134 Jack Nicholson, *Vanity Fair*, April 1994

137 Cynthia Heimel, *Untamed Tongues: Wild Words from Wild Women* (Conari Press, 1993)

141 Christopher Hampton, *The Fifth and Far Finer Than the First Four 637 Best Things Anybody Ever Said* (Ballantine Books, 1993)

144 Nora Ephron, *Untamed Tongues: Wild Words from Wild Women* (Conari Press, 1993)

146 Susan Powter, *Stop the Insanity!* (Simon & Schuster, 1993)

156–57 Walt Whitman, *21st Century Dictionary of Quotations* (Dell Publishing, 1993)

159 Ludwig Wittgenstein, *Philosophical Investigations*, 1953

162–63 Duke of Windsor, *Just Joking*, portions by Donald L. Smith, portions by Jon Winokur (WordStar International, 1992)

170 Monica Piper, *Just Joking*, portions by Donald L. Smith, portions by Jon Winokur (WordStar International, 1992)

174 Oscar Wilde, *1,911 Best Things Anybody Ever Said* (Ballantine Books, 1988)

180–81 Betty Friedan, *The Fountain of Age* (Simon & Schuster, 1993)

183 Ellen DeGeneres, *Just Joking*, portions by Donald L. Smith, portions by Jon Winokur (WordStar International, 1992)

185 *Sleeper*, 1973

190 Jack Kevorkian, *Vanity Fair*, July 1994

192 Anaïs Nin, *The Quotable Quote Book: Wisecracks, Wit & Wisdom of the Current Times*, by Merrit Malloy and Shauna Sorensen (Citadel Press, 1990)

192 Nikos Kazantzakis, *Zorba the Greek*, (Simon & Schuster, 1953)

193 Sigmund Freud, *21st Century Dictionary of Quotations* (Dell Publishing, 1993)

195 Dr. Gonzo, *1,911 Best Things Anybody Ever Said* (Ballantine Books, 1988)

196 Coco Chanel, *The Last Word: A Treasury of Women's Quotes*, by Carolyn Warner (Prentice-Hall, 1992)

197 Polish proverb, *Forbes*, January 4, 1992

198 Dolly Parton, quoted in *San Francisco Chronicle*, December 31, 1984, *The Last Word: A Treasury of Women's Quotes*, by Carolyn Warner (Prentice-Hall, 1992)

199 Luigi Pirandello, *The Rules of the Game*, 1918

200 Eugène Ionesco, *Peter's Quotations* (Morrow, 1977)

201 Raymond Chandler, *The Penguin Book of Modern Humorous Quotations* (Penguin Books, 1987)

202 Orson Welles, *Newsweek*, July 30, 1973

203 Will Rogers, *21st Century Dictionary of Quotations* (Dell Publishing, 1993)

204 Ronnie Shakes, *Just Joking*, portions by Donald L. Smith, portions by Jon Winokur (WordStar International, 1992)

206 John Mendoza, *Just Joking*, portions by Donald L. Smith, portions by Jon Winokur (WordStar International, 1992)

207 Jacques Bénigne, *Correct Quotes*, portions by Career Publishing (WordStar International, 1992)

208 Liz Winston, *The Fifth and Far Finer Than the First Four 637 Best Things Anybody Ever Said* (Ballantine Books, 1993)

210 Susie Bright, quoted in *Talk Dirty to Me* by Sallie Tisdale (Doubleday, 1994)

210 Steve Martin, *Just Joking*, portions by Donald L. Smith, portions by Jon Winokur (WordStar International, 1992)

211 Jack Lemmon, *Some Like It Hot*

211 Merrill Markoe, *NY Woman*, November 1991

213 Friedrich Nietzsche, *21st Century Dictionary of Quotations* (Dell Publishing, 1993)

213 Jane Wagner, *The Quotable Quote Book: Wisecracks, Wit & Wisdom of the Current Times* by Merrit Malloy and Shauna Sorensen (Citadel Press, 1990)

224 Robert Browning, *Forbes*, October 26, 1992

ACKNOWLEDGMENTS

MANUFACTURER & RETAIL RESEARCH Jeannette Durkan
QUOTE RESEARCH Kate Doyle Hooper & Lige Rushing
FIRST AID RESEARCH & TEXT CONTRIBUTION Deborah Freeman
ORIGINAL INTERVIEWS Cynthia Stuart
CASTING AGENT Jill Glover

MODELS Wale Agbaje, Alan Cresto, Tim Daniels, Derek, John Foster, John Francis, Marinda Hanselmann, Marieme, Maggie O'Brien, Lorraine Pasquale, Sergio, Farrah Summerford, Janey Tomba, Rosie Vela, Travis C. Waller, Lisa Wolf, Susan Zabrowski.

AND SPECIAL THANKS TO Connie Bang, Amy Capen, Tony Chirico, Jin Chung, Jill Cohen, Lauri Del Commune, Dovanna, Michael Drazen, Dr. Nelson Freeman, Jane Friedman, Janice Goldklang, Dr. Robert Greenburg, Torkil Gudnason, Dina Dell'Arciprete Houser, Patrick Higgins, Ray Hooper, Kimie Horikoshi, Katherine Hourigan, Andy Hughes, Carol Janeway, Barbara Jones-Diggs, Mikako Koyama, Dr. Jerome Lahman, Nicholas Latimer, Carl Lennertz, Dr. Gila Lighter, William Loverd, Anne McCormick, Dwyer McIntosh, Sonny Mehta, Anne Messitte, Yasuhiro Mizoi, Ted Muehling, Joseph Muniz, Lan Nguyen, Cathy O'Brien, Linda Philips, Dr. Robert Rodner, Dr. Joseph Segal, Anne-Lise Spitzer, Shelley Wanger, Mark Weiss, Amy Zenn.

CHIC SIMPLE STAFF
MOM AND DAD Kim & Jeff
OFFICE MANAGER Jo-Anne Harrison
ART DIRECTOR Wayne Wolf
DESIGN/PRODUCTION M. Scott Cookson, Aileen Tse
RESEARCH Deborah Freeman
COPY EDITOR Borden Elniff

COMMUNICATIONS

The world has gotten smaller and faster but we still can only be in one place at a time, which is why we are anxious to hear from you. We would like your input on stores and products that have impressed you. We are always happy to answer any questions you have about items in the book, and of course we are interested in feedback about Chic Simple.

Our address is: **84 WOOSTER STREET NEW YORK, NY 10012**
Fax: **(212) 343-9678**
Compuserve number: 72704,2346
email address: **info@chicsimple.com**

Stay in touch because . . .
"The more you know, the less you need."

KIM JOHNSON GROSS & JEFF STONE

A NOTE ON THE TYPE

The text of this book was set in two typefaces: New Baskerville and Futura. The ITC version of **NEW BASKERVILLE** is called Baskerville, which itself is a facsimile reproduction of types cast from molds made by John Baskerville (1706–1775) from his designs. Baskerville's original face was one of the forerunners of the typestyle known to printers as the "modern face"—a "modern" of the period A.D. 1800. **FUTURA** was produced in 1928 by Paul Renner (1878–1956), former director of the Munich School of Design, for the Bauer Type Foundry. Futura is simple in design and wonderfully restful in reading. It has been widely used in advertising because of its even, modern appearance in mass and its harmony with a great variety of other modern types.

SEPARATION AND FILM PREPARATION BY

DIGITAL COLOR ASSOCIATES, INC.
Hauppauge, New York

PRINTED AND BOUND BY

R. R. DONNELLEY & SONS
Willard, Ohio

HARDWARE

Apple Macintosh Quadra 700 and 800 personal computers; APS Technologies Syquest Drives; MicroNet DAT Drive; SuperMac 21" Color Monitor; Radius PrecisionColor Display/20; Radius 24X series Video Board; Hewlett-Packard LaserJet 4, Supra Fax Modem

SOFTWARE

QuarkXPress 3.3, Adobe Photoshop 2.5.1, Microsoft Word 5.1, FileMaker Pro 2.0, Adobe Illustrator 5.0.1

MUSICWARE

Nirvana (*In Utero*), Jimi Hendrix (*The Ultimate Experience*), Deep Forest, Miles Davis (*Kind of Blue*), Cocteau Twins (*Four-Calendar Café*), Marvin Gaye (*Anthology*), the Breeders (*Last Splash*), Pearl Jam, Ali Farka Toure with Ry Cooder (*Talking Timbuktu*), Bill Morrissey (*Night Train*), Lucky Dube (*Victims*), *Bird: The Complete Charlie Parker on Verve* (Discs 1–4), Radiohead (*Pablo Honey*), Hildegard of Bingen (*A Feather on the Breath of God*), Merle Haggard (*Chill Factor*), Duke Ellington (*Solos, Duets and Trios*), Chris Rea (*Espresso Logic*), Angélique Kidjo (*Ayé*), AFX (*Analogue Bubblebath*), *The Acid Jazz Text Part 1*, Chet Baker (*My Funny Valentine*), Black Uhuru (*Mystical Truth Dub*), An English Ladymass (*Medieval Chant and Polyphony*), Milt Jackson and John Coltrane (*Bags & Trane*), *The Very Best of Moby Grape* (Vintage), Stan Getz (*The Best of the Verve Years, Volume 1*), *Bluesiana Hot Sauce*, Mokum (*F**king Hardcore*), Elvis Costello (*Brutal Youth*).

"If you get simple beauty, and naught else, you get about the best thing God invents."

ROBERT BROWNING